SECRETS TO EFFECTIVE
PAIN MANAGEMENT

By Jeffrey C. Bado, D.O.

This book is dedicated to my chronic pain patients who changed my life by sharing their experiences and teaching me how to effectively treat chronic pain.

TABLE OF CONTENTS

Introduction

Welcome to the First Edition of "Secrets to Effective Pain Management." This book is an anthology of my web posts on various topics on pain management. My website chronicpainreliefoptions.com is a blog site where I write about topics of interest for my readers regarding pain syndromes, pain treatments, and controversies in pain management. Over the past many months, it became evident that many of my readers would appreciate an expanded form of what I post on my website. It was their interest in my blog site that was the inspiration for this book.

This book is an amalgam of my 26 years as a practicing physician. I was the "reluctant" pain management physician. The entry into the field of Pain Management was neither an initial interest of mine nor a vision for my career. My initial training in medicine was as an Internal Medicine specialist. Doctors who practice Internal Medicine are the "clinical detectives" of the medical profession. We are supposed to think of diagnoses where most Doctors would not. The popular medical TV show called, "House" is about such an Internist. My early practice of medicine was entirely devoted to the discovery and management of diverse diseases. I am naturally most suited to such an endeavor.

But God had different plans for me. Over the years, I encountered many patients who lived with chronic pain. Most of these poor souls were not being effectively treated for their chronic pain syndromes. At first my venture into Pain Management was confined to a few people with terminal illnesses. Even at the end of their lives, with intractable and excruciating pain, they could not seem to find a Pain Management Doctor that would effectively treat their pain. As their Internist, I was thrust into the responsibility of doing so out of compassion.

There was no time or mechanism for me to enter a formal Pain Management program for training. I was in active medical practice, had a family to provide for, and medical education debt to pay back. So I began to read, attend conferences, and most of all...listen to my patients teach me what was the most effective way to treat pain. As an Internist, I had been taught how to think critically and discern truth. My patient's comments about their pain care rang true to me. My education in pain management could be called, "self-taught."

The need for pain management became obvious as more and more people presented to my practice with undertreated chronic pain. I did not advertise or market myself as a Pain Management expert initially. However, my perspective on the field evolved in a way that it would not have if I had been formally trained in a structured Pain Management program. Although I learned most of the topics that any formally trained Pain Management Doctor would have in an official program, there was a fundamental difference in my "training." It was patient centered.

The primary source of the effectiveness of the pain therapies came directly from patients. What better source of truth could I have? Who would know better what worked than a patient in pain? To that knowledge, through experience, I added the academic information to buttress the science side of things. I believe that type of "training" is the most effective. My patients taught me how so many of the procedures that were used as primary therapy for pain did not work (or gave very temporary pain relief). They even taught me how some pain doctors leveraged the more profitable surgical procedures by giving ineffective doses of opiate pain medications (sometimes actually telling a patient they would not get their pain medications if they did not have the surgical procedure). This is an unethical practice in my opinion.

Pain doctors have been given the "green light" to prefer profitable procedures over an effective practice. The likelihood of legal reprisal for ineffective surgical procedures over effective opiate therapy is less (certainly criminal indictment is less). Given the options, it is understandable why the minimally useful practice of spinal injections for chronic pain has become so popular. The pain patients find themselves caught in the middle. They can even become financial commodities welcomed in interventional pain practices until their medical insurance no longer pays for the expensive procedures.

I discovered the growing need to serve the patient population that was underinsured or uninsured. It was this population that my pain practice focused upon. In time, I also saw that my practice would eventually not meet the need of the pain patients either. There was another need in Pain Management, that being, the need for the chronic pain patient to transition to self-care. Thus, the creation of my website and this book were created to present ideas for how you can relieve your own pain. In most cases, you will want to have this supervised by your Pain Management practitioner. I simply want to facilitate you to manage your own case and make you less dependent on a Pain Management clinician. Over my 26 years of practice, I found that the patients who do so will eventually find relief of their pain and a greater measure of autonomy.

The advice in this book has been tested in clinical practice. This is not a theoretical book. Here again, this is because the advice in this book is what my patients have told me. It is people like yourself who have really contributed the content that I share with you. Their voices are speaking to you through this book. They understood your pain as they owned their own. You will want to listen to what they are saying to you.

This book can also be used as a resource for suggestions to the clinician supervising your pain management. It is not meant as an authoritative text for you to independently diagnose and treat your chronic pain. This book will give insights into chronic pain that you will find in no other book. Again, that is because it is a reflection of pain management from the patient's point of view. By my estimate, there is no other book like it available to you.

You can read each section separately or read through the book in its entirety. Either method will prove valuable to you. When read in its entirety you will see a pattern that emerges for the best way to diagnose and treat chronic pain. That pattern emphasizes the value of the complete history and physical (which has been largely replaced by diagnostic studies with today's high tech emphasis). You will also notice many advantages and limitations to diagnostic testing.

The approach to establishing the main mechanism for the generation of pain in any given syndrome is also unique (a neuro-matrix approach). By establishing the central neuro-mechanism for your chronic pain, a clinician will be better able to construct an effective treatment regimen. A diagnosis is often not enough. The mechanism explains the actual physiology involved in generating a certain type of pain. This functional approach avoids the natural tendency for a physician to use a "recipe" or "protocol" approach to medical care. It will cause the treating physician to individualize the treatment plan for each patient.

Every human being is unique. There are no two alike...even with identical twins. The same diagnosis in different people will require individualization of the treatment plan. Your pain is unique to you and you deserve special consideration for its relief. I think you will find some practical advice on the following pages. Think of this book as a continual work in progress. I hope you will give me some feedback, suggestions, and criticisms so I can upgrade the Second Edition. Feel free to contact me via epiduraldoc1982@gmail.com. Enjoy the book.

Wishing you joy and healing,

Jeffrey C. Bado, D.O.

Chapter 1 – Secrets about the Differences Between Acute and Chronic Pain

- Peripheral Neuropathy
- Fibromyalgia (FMS)
- Thyroid Issues
- Insulin Resistance (metabolic syndrome)
- Syndrome X/Pre-diabetes
- Vertigo
- Sciatica
- CF Syndrome
- Chronic Back or Neck Pain
- Stenosis
- IBS
- Insomnia
- Crohn's Disease
- Celiac
- PCOS/Infertility
- Migranes/Chronic Headaches
- ADD/ADHD
- Autism Spectrum Disorder
- Symptoms of MS, MD
- Stroke

- O2 Deficits (Anemias)
- Neurological Misfiring
- Metabolic Imbalances
- Blood sugar Imbalances
- Cortisol Imbalances
- Hormonal Imbalances
- Auto-immune Imbalances
- Immune Imbalances
- Food Sensitivities
- Brain Imbalances

All are conditions of neurological, metabolic, and musculoskeletal imbalances.

Medical model vs functional model

Chronic pain is any daily pain that persists for 3 or more months. Did you know that the vast majority of medical practitioners in practice today did not receive any unique training in chronic pain?

This is why there is so much controversy about the treatment of it. Most practitioners have very adequate training in acute pain (pain that lasts less than 3 months). Acute pain is an early warning system that tells you that there is a problem. Without acute pain, you would not know that you have a health problem and need to see your primary care practitioner (PCP).

Secret Number 1: The Chronic Pain Syndrome is a completely different syndrome from Acute Pain with different mechanisms and different therapies.

The Chronic Pain Syndrome changes your nervous system, affects your metabolism, impairs your immune system, and can even cause depression in people who are not prone to it (see the above chart). The Chronic Pain Syndrome lacks some of the other associated physical findings that acute pain has (sweating, rapid heart rate, etc.). Also, if a person suffers from the Chronic Pain Syndrome they have a higher risk of other diseases (whereas acute pain does not increase your risk of other diseases). So why would a Doctor tell a person with chronic pain that they must just, "live with it?"

Secret Number 2: It is important to treat chronic pain as effectively as possible as soon as possible.

Untreated chronic pain can result in changes in your central nervous system, endocrine system, and immune system that are deleterious to your health. These changes may become permanent. **Untreated chronic pain increases death from a variety of other illnesses too (such as heart disease, stroke, and cancer).**

Thus, the Chronic Pain Syndrome is a disease all unto itself. This is a very important distinction from acute pain. It can cause confusion among PCPs who have not been trained in chronic pain (which is most Doctors). So...if you are suffering from chronic pain you need to do several things. First, you must make sure you have had an accurate history, physical, and diagnostic workup for your pain. If your PCP is unable to do this, you will need to be referred to a specialist.

Secret Number 3: You will know that you have had an adequate workup when your PCP can give you a precise diagnosis and tell you the neuro-mechanism for your chronic pain.

 A team of specialists may need to be gathered to construct a treatment regimen that targets the mechanism for your chronic pain. You will encounter several challenges with this as it is expensive and time-consuming. If your pain is not relieved within 6 months, most insurance companies will begin to limit paying for your care. In most cases of chronic pain, the responsibility will eventually fall to the individual in pain to construct their own treatment regimen.

Remember, relief of your pain will take some time. Unlike acute pain, chronic pain has caused changes in your body that can only be reversed through chronic therapy. This will usually take 6 or more weeks to work. You have to prepare yourself for a long journey. This is very challenging when you have been hurting for many months already.

There is hope that you can achieve a radical improvement in your Chronic Pain Syndrome if you follow these basic guidelines. You do not have to despair...hope is a reality if you take charge of your own pain relief. This book has been particularly written for that person who has experienced chronic pain and feels as if there is no other alternative but to "live with it." There is hope if you follow the guidelines that you will read in the various chapters that follow.

Chapter 2 – Secrets to the Approach of the Person with Chronic Pain

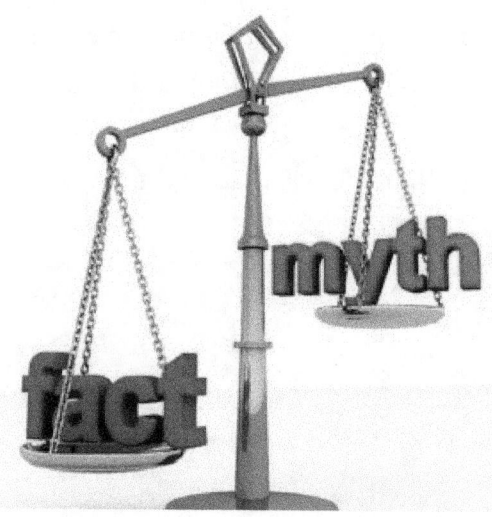

If you are suffering from chronic pain (or a loved one is suffering), you must realize that your body is always changing. Even if you were initially well controlled on your medication or with the pain relieving therapies, you could expect your body will adapt.

Change does not necessarily mean that your pain syndrome will worsen. Over 26 years of medical practice showed me that most people will get better on a well-planned treatment regimen while only a few will get worse. However, no one stays the same. Even with an accurate diagnosis and optimal therapy you may worsen. That does not necessarily mean that you are doing anything wrong (or your Doctor for that matter). It is just the way things can work. It is Physics...everything goes to greater and greater disorganization (called entropy). Wrinkles are a manifestation of this process (as is other body parts that sag).

Yet and still, I had most of my patients improve. Over time their slower acting medications actually reversed the neural pain processing that was mediating their discomfort. In some cases, my patients made radical lifestyle changes that resulted in the reduction of their chronic pain. Change can be positive too.

You may be asking, "What could it mean if my pain is getting worse?" I see at least seven secrets for why this happens in people:

Secret Number 1: The underlying disease process has worsened.

The most common reason for worsening of chronic pain is the unrelenting progression of the disease process that caused the pain to begin with. For instance, the most common cause of low back pain is Osteoarthritis (OA). OA is really a "wearing out" of joints, ligaments, and tendons.

It would make sense that the process would continue as long as you are alive.

To be certain, the process ends with death. In an odd sort of way, the progression of OA is reflective of being alive. Because a person is diagnosed at a point in time with OA does not mean that there would not be progression. Most diseases are like this...consider heart disease. The likelihood of a second heart attack is greater than with the first (also true with strokes). This is because the process that caused the heart disease to begin with has continued. You will want to institute the measures necessary to slow down or stop the main disease process that is causing your chronic pain.

Secret Number 2: Your activity level has increased requiring an increase in your therapy.

Sometimes the pain management is so effective that a patient actually increases their activity level. Of course, one should then expect that their requirements for pain medicine would increase. I had patients that were able to return to work when placed on effective pain management. They usually required an increase in their medicine with the increase in work activity. Does this make sense to you? If you drive your automobile with a "heavy foot" your brakes will require more frequent maintenance and your oil changes will too. Again, it is simple physics.

Secret Number 3: Your body has adapted to the therapy.

Your body is in a never ending state of readjustment. Things that are high will eventually come low and vice versa. It is called a "negative feedback loop." It is essential for the efficiency of the physiology of the body. It is what body builders rely on for the massive gains in muscle they achieve. Your entire body chemistry relies on this process for efficient function.

The medicines and procedures that you may utilize for pain relief may also become ineffective over time. The body adjusts naturally. The medications and procedures haven't changed...you have. It is expected that your requirement for pain medicine will increase over time. This is not addiction. Most people need a change in their dose or type of medicine every 12 to 24 months' even if they initially were well balanced on their medications.

Secret Number 4: You have developed additional causes for your pain.

While the primary cause of your chronic pain will likely remain, the rest of your body is subject to other destructive influences over time. Even if you were able to radically modify the primary mechanism causing your pain you may develop a second or third mechanism. This is often because the systems that were not originally dysfunctional have had additional stress put upon them. For instance, paraplegics (people with paralyzed legs) often develop Carpal Tunnel Syndrome of their wrists due to the additional weight burden placed on their arms moving their entire body weight.

Secret Number 5: You are on inadequate doses of pain medicine or are receiving inadequate therapy.

The nervous system is constantly changing in response to internal and external stimuli. This is called neuroplasticity. Nerves become more efficient at conducting pain impulses if they are continuously stimulated. Under treating pain can not only worsen the primary mechanism for a person's pain but will enhance the ability to perceive and transmit the pain. This is called, "wind-up." It has been shown in experimental studies that compared subjects undertreated for their level of pain with those properly treated. Ultimately, those inadequately treated do much worse that people properly treated at the outset of their pain syndrome when each had the same diagnosis. Early adequate treatment of chronic pain reduces "wind-up" and the other negative physiologic changes with chronic pain. The old adage, "just live with it" has been debunked with more recent scientific studies (though old habits with Doctors die slowly in medicine).

Secret Number 6: You are on the wrong medicine or have received the wrong therapy.

All primary mechanisms for pain are not the same. Neuropathic pain is treated with different medications from inflammatory pain. Though opiate pain medications are effective for most types of pain, the challenging side effects make them a category of medication that will always be controversial to use. *In any case, identification of the primary neuro-mechanism for a pain syndrome is essential for initiating and maintaining the best therapy.* In my practice of pain management, I rarely saw patients who had a good explanation given to them for the primary mechanism of their pain. If a patient doesn't understand the main reason for their pain, they will be less invested in the therapy. Furthermore, they will not be able to knowledgeably adjust their therapy regimen between visits...a situation that makes the chronic pain patient very dependent on their medical providers.

Secret Number 7: You have become addicted to your pain medicines.

Finally, the consideration of addiction is warranted in people who take their medications so erratically that they could develop bodily harm from doing so. This is a most challenging aspect of pain management as most addicts do not honestly report their non-compliance. Even in the most compliant patients, only 60% of patients will actually take their medications as directed. Human beings are imperfect as a species and require a great deal of encouragement.

I do not believe that vilification of Doctor or patient will have the best result. Our present system has created an adversarial relationship between the parties involved. It must change. If you find that your pain management is not meeting your pain needs, you will need a re-evaluation. My bias is for that to be done by a Doctor, who believes in a "primary neuro-mechanism for pain" approach (a functional approach). I do not believe that most pain Doctors actually mentally process this way. It would appear that most pain Doctors take a more diagnosis oriented approach to pain management. We spend billions of dollars on pain management yearly in the U. S. and the American public is not "getting their money's worth." Many aspects of pain management need to improve: the legal system needs to change its criminalization approach to the addict, doctors must stand up for their patients and advocate for them, insurance companies need to finance only what works, and patients need to take more responsibility for their healthcare.

As I close this chapter let me remind you...I never met a patient with chronic pain that I was unable to reduce their discomfort. After establishing the primary mechanism for their pain, I was always able to construct a treatment regimen that would work. The purpose of this book is to teach you the "secrets" to this approach. If you or a loved one is experiencing pain, you will have a reduction in pain...hope is your reality. No one's pain is "too severe" to be beyond relief.

Chapter 3 – The Secret Characteristic That Must Be Evident In the Doctors Who Treat Chronic Pain

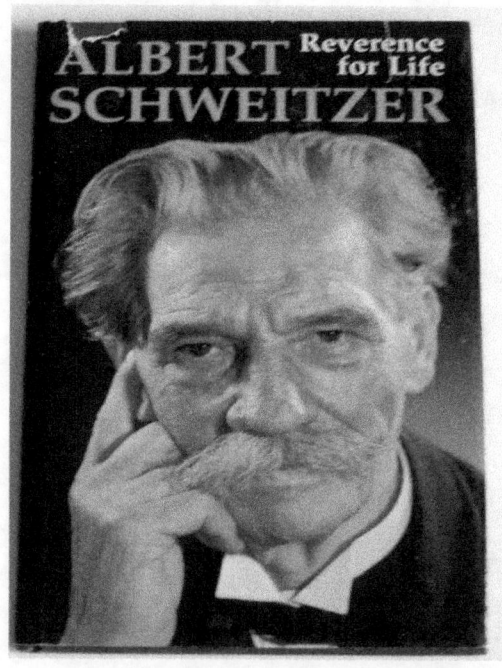

In this chapter, I am going to explain the "secret" characteristic that a Pain Management physician must have to be effective in reducing their patient's pain.

I never wondered what I was going to do with my life. I knew that becoming a physician was what I was "called" to do. I knew the qualities of a good doctor because I was cared for by one. The fee for his services seemed so small in comparison to the comfort he gave us whenever we needed his care. I made the decision to be a doctor at the age of 6 years old and dedicated my life to helping others until my retirement. My marriage and my family paid the price for me being the doctor I thought I should be. Being a doctor was never a job...it was a calling.

Nearly every family doctor in my small hometown of Kenmore, New York made house calls. The mere presence of our doctor at our bedside was enough to know that you would be ok. And yet, in the 1950s, the treatments were limited. There were several antibiotics, a few high blood pressure medications, and even fewer cancer treatments. The average American male lived to be 67 years-old in 1955. My maternal grandfather "lived a full life" and died at 55 years old (I was four at the time). He owned several homes, worked two jobs, did life insurance sales in the evenings, and helped build our little Hungarian church. He also suffered from chronic back pain from working on my great-grandfather's farm (now a state park outside Niagara Falls, New York).

Our first family doctor was given a loan by my maternal grandfather (MGF) so he could go to medical school (they were both Hungarian immigrants). His younger brother also went to medical school on my MGF. The Hungarians stuck together in those days. We knew that Doctors weren't perfect people. There were misdiagnoses and delayed diagnoses all the time. Even then, we all knew that our Doctor had our best interest at heart. It was impossible for any human being to know everything. He was still just a man. His perfection was not what we believed in...it was him. His heart...his dedication...his empathy for us is what we admired most about our doctor.

I grew up on the doctor television shows "Dr. Kildare" and "Dr. Ben Casey." I can still remember Dr. Zorba's words (he was the wise mentor for Dr. Casey, a brilliant surgeon in the series). In the introduction to nearly every episode of "Ben Casey," he was to be shown giving a lecture. In that lecture scene to the hospital Interns (Doctors in training), Dr. Zorba drew symbols on a chalkboard and said, "Man...woman...birth...death...infinity..." I was 6 years-old and recall it like it was yesterday. The summary of an entire human life in 5 words by Dr. Zorba. Doctors were to understand the foibles of human beings. We respected our doctors and did not expect perfection. Our health was our primary responsibility. Perhaps only in the case of gross misconduct would we ever consider a legal action against a doctor. He was our protector, advocate, and friend.

American's feelings about Doctors began to change along with our society. We "lost our innocence" as a culture when President Kennedy was assassinated under circumstances that have never been properly explained. The civil rights movement followed along with a war in Vietnam that we have never completely healed from. The attitudes of people toward authority figures they trusted began to change. Skepticism devolved to cynicism. We began to wonder whether our leaders related to the American people.

I went to medical school in 1978. Being accepted into medical school was still a privilege. It was not the medical school's benefit to have me attend their school. It was mine. Despite my hard work to get in, there was no feeling of entitlement. They didn't owe me...I owed them...and I paid them handsomely for that privilege. I went to medical school wanting to be Dr. Ben Casey. I didn't consider the prospects of malpractice, malpractice insurance, local regulations, state regulations, federal regulations, insurance company intrusion, nor the cynical media scourge of physicians.

In just 8 years, the medical profession changed in the mind of the public from a noble one to a group of intellectual elites (some profit driven) that was detached from the plight of their patients. And yet, I was doing house calls, was on call 24 hours a day for my patients, did hospital rounds at 3 hospitals, and was paying off my medical school debt until I retired. And I was not alone...many of the doctors I knew did the same thing. We also had more medications, better diagnostic equipment, and more cures than had ever occurred in the history of medicine. Yet, the schism between doctors and patients widened ever more.

Most doctors today are on the defensive. I know of practices that do background checks on new patients before admitting them to their practice. They are looking for evidence of previous lawsuits against other physicians. Those practices will expel any patient they deem as "lawsuit prone." But isn't the health of patients better than ever? Just look at the life expectancy of the average American today. As of 2010 the average American male could be expected to live to 76 years-old and average American female to 81 years of age. We perform millions of life-saving surgeries each year in the U.S., have eradicated polio, decreased the lethality of pneumonia, are close to curing many previously incurable diseases (consider AIDS for one), and are the number one country in the world for research.

And yet, recent Gallup polls show that more Americans are unhappy with their medical care than ever. The relationship between doctor and patient continues to be strained by forces that are mostly outside of direct medical care. The Doctor – patient relationship has been damaged.

I give you that historical backdrop and behind the scenes look like a foundation for what I am about to tell you. Whether you believe it or not...you, as a patient, can change this relationship deterioration. That sounds radical doesn't it? However, you need to know that the real power to upgrade the Doctor – patient relationship is largely up to you. There will be no law, or lawyer, or insurance company, or any other inducement separate and apart from the patients themselves, that will improve doctor - patient relationships.

What do you think is the most important characteristic your pain doctor must have to be able to do the best for you? The quality I am going to share is so important that if your pain Doctor doesn't have it you shouldn't just walk away from their practice...you need to run. Is it a high intellect?   The profession is full of cold geniuses. Is it vast knowledge? The profession is brimming over with limitless egos. Is it elite training? Every training institution has its deficiencies for there is no perfect educational system. Every doctor eventually encounters a case where their training is insufficient.

There is one characteristic that, in my opinion, is the most important of all. Without this characteristic fully developed in your Doctor, there is no intellect, knowledge, or training program that can ever compensate for it. ***The secret characteristic that must be evident in all Doctors who treat chronic pain is empathy.*** Empathy is the experience of understanding another person's condition from their perspective. An empathic Doctor would never allow their intellect to rule them. It would never allow their knowledge to inflate them. Empathy will even create a humility that puts a limit on how confident a doctor is in their training. They would ask for help more readily. When I was applying to medical school, I was never asked one question in my interviews about empathy. It is not emphasized in medical school entrance qualifications to this day. As a teacher of physicians, I met too many young doctors who lacked empathy. The error is compounding.

All the great positive social evolutionaries (notice I didn't say revolutionaries) such as Moses, Jesus, Gandhi, Martin Luther King, and Mother Teresa were great empaths. It is the one quality that Doctors must have to qualify as a Pain Management specialist. Chronic pain does not have a technical device to measure its existence. All of the diagnostic studies evaluate structure or function of the human body. Doctors must rely on the testimony of their patients for the existence of pain. You could no more tell the temperature of an oven by simply looking at it than you can tell how much pain a person is in by simply looking at them. Empathy gives the Doctor the capacity to "feel the pain" of his/her patients.

In this chapter, I have reviewed how the relationship between patients and Doctors has changed. Americans are less contented with their Doctors than they have ever been despite all the medical advances. I believe this has been the result of medical training neglecting the need for a physician to have empathy for their patients as an essential personality characteristic.   As a patient, you must find a pain Doctor that understands your perspective. Make it an uncompromising requirement that your Doctor relates with you and your pain. All the other aspects of being a good Doctor are subservient to this characteristic. The empathy of your Pain Management provider has the power to transform your life. An empathic physician will lead to a transcendent relationship. Your pain relief will become your reality.

Chapter 4 – Secrets of the Neurophysiology of Pain

Neuromatrix Theory of Pain

- Theory that the matrix of neurons in the brain is capable of generating pain (and other sensations) in the absence of signals from sensory nerves.

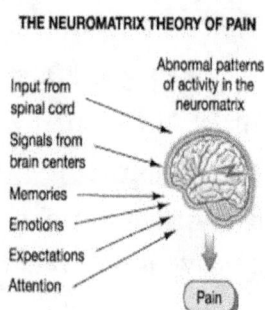

THE NEUROMATRIX THEORY OF PAIN

Input from spinal cord

Signals from brain centers

Memories

Emotions

Expectations

Attention

Abnormal patterns of activity in the neuromatrix

Pain

The explanation for how people actually feel pain is evolving. The process of peripheral generation of a pain stimulus, transduction, transmission, translation, and perception of pain is well taught in medical schools. This actual process was originally described by Rene Descartes in 1633. He was a philosopher who originally developed the Cartesian approach to pain. It essentially begins with tissue damage as the pain generator which is changed into an electrical neural signal (transduction). The signal is then conducted (transmission) and processed throughout the brain network (translation) so that the final understanding of the pain results in the frontal lobes of the brain (perception).

This approach works well for explaining acute pain but has many shortcomings with understanding chronic pain. For instance, it would not explain the phenomena of "Phantom Pain" (see chapter 6) where pain persists long after tissue damage has healed. In fact, the "Phantom Pain" is actually perceived in a body part that no longer exists (such as experiencing pain where a hand used to exist). Even low back pain can exist where there is little diagnostic evidence of tissue damage.

To further challenge the Cartesian approach to pain, there are many people who have severe abnormalities of structure but no pain. There are countless examples of people with abnormal MRIs of their lumbar spine who have little or no pain. This approach falls short again in explaining how pain is not perceived in an obviously tissue damaged state. Despite this inconsistency in the Cartesian approach to pain, many Pain Physicians rely on this approach to explain their patient's pain. If a diagnostic study does not show structural abnormalities that support the patient's symptoms, the patient is often labeled a malingerer.

As you will see over and over in this book, a more comprehensive approach must be used when explaining the chronic pain. Pain is a central nervous system phenomenon. The spinal cord and brain (the central nervous system) don't just receive the pain stimulus from tissue damage; they create and modify it. Previous learning, attention, mental disposition, neurotransmitter levels, receptor types-levels-distribution, hormonal levels, relationships with microglial cells, etc. all affect the generation of pain. In this book, my mantra will be to ask the question, "What is the neuro-mechanism for pain generation?" This not only could include tissue damage but all the other central nervous system mechanisms. My approach emphasizes neuro-matrix over an actual tissue damage diagnosis. This approach adequately explains all the pain disorders, both those with identifiable tissue damage and those without apparent tissue damage.

Unfortunately, the Cartesian approach is still held by most physicians (especially interventional pain management physicians). Old habits die hard in medicine. Tradition is often held in higher esteem than new facts. The pressure placed on Pain Management physicians to have "objective" reasons for pain in a patient (a diagnostic study instead of the opinion of a Doctor) has caused the Cartesian approach to persist too. Administering opiate pain medications to a patient without an "objective study" can lead a Doctor to criminal charges. This happens in spite of literature to the contrary. And yet, all diagnostic studies require interpretation by a human being (usually a Doctor) which begs the question, "Are diagnostic studies truly objective?"

Since pain is a neurophysiologic phenomenon, measuring a structural abnormality to gauge pain does not make sense. At the present, there is no clinical diagnostic study that measures pain. This means that a Pain Management physician must always rely on the testimony of their patient to know whether pain actually exists. Relying on a structural test to reveal whether pain exists or not is akin to looking at your oven and being able to tell the temperature of it. Obviously, a functional measurement of temperature is the only way to know how hot the oven is. There is no comparative diagnostic study for pain.

Dr. Melzack could be considered the first pain management expert to evoke the neuro-matrix model of pain. In 1965, Dr. Melzack (along with Dr. Wall) published an article which explained the "Gate Theory" of pain. In that article, the notion that the central nervous system (CNS) was the source of all pain was first advanced. By "closing the gate" for pain transmission in the spinal cord pain could be completely stopped (independent of on-going tissue damage). In later articles Dr. Melzack was able to explain many diverse pain syndromes that the Cartesian model could not. The idea that all pain is created in the CNS was novel.

In summary, the neurophysiology of pain always includes the generation of pain signaling in the CNS. Where possible, a peripheral pain generator should also be treated. The approach to each pain syndrome should begin with what is happening mechanistically at the level of the CNS. A reasonable search for a peripheral pain generator should then be pursued. However, failing to find a peripheral generator does not immediately assume the pain is fictitious. The treatment of any given pain syndrome should begin with the central mechanism while doing a reasonable search for a peripheral generator. As you read in this book, you will see this approach to chronic pain has application to all syndromes. The effect of its application can yield stunning reductions in chronic pain.

Chapter 5 – Secrets of Common Chronic Pain Disorders

I. Chronic Low Back Pain Secrets

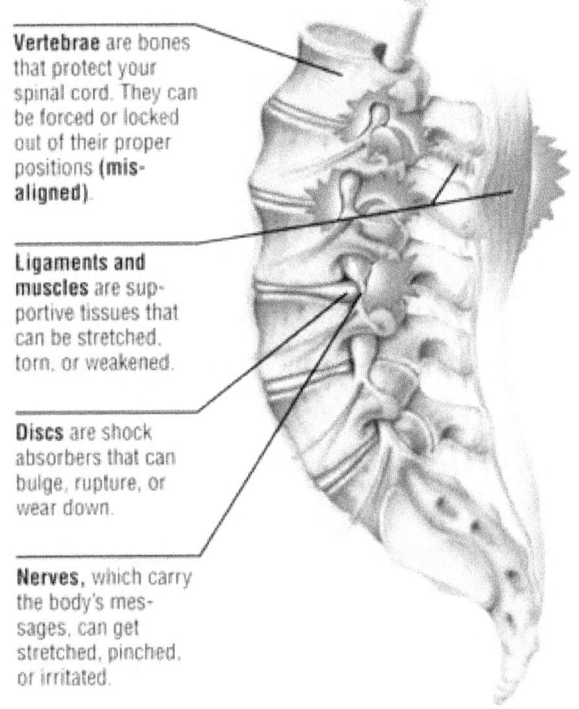

Vertebrae are bones that protect your spinal cord. They can be forced or locked out of their proper positions (**mis-aligned**).

Ligaments and muscles are supportive tissues that can be stretched, torn, or weakened.

Discs are shock absorbers that can bulge, rupture, or wear down.

Nerves, which carry the body's messages, can get stretched, pinched, or irritated.

One of the leading causes of pain and disability in the U.S. is chronic low back pain (pain that is continuous for over 3 months). Just as in other causes of chronic pain, knowing the neuro-mechanism (the actual way in which the pain is generated) is essential to achieving relief. Most people with chronic pain have not had the correct neuro-mechanism for their pain identified.

Secret Number 1: Chronic low back pain is usually due to one or more of 3 different mechanisms: 1) a muscular problem and/or 2) a skeletal problem and/or 3) a neural (nerve) problem.

It really isn't more complicated than that. The problem is that a proper history, physical, or diagnostic workup has usually not been done before assigning a diagnosis. Once you have the correct diagnosis, there are many effective treatments that can be employed. **When the cause of the chronic low back pain seems to mysteriously elude the doctor, it is usually something simple that has not been done.** Your body makes sense and follows certain general rules.

Secret Number 2: Securing an accurate diagnosis and neuro-mechanism makes the treatments very straightforward.

A muscular problem needs to have the blood flow to the muscle enhanced so as to promote healing. A skeletal problem needs to have the spine aligned (straightened) and stretched. A neural problem needs to facilitate healing of the peripheral nerve and normalization of central nervous system pain generation.

Remember...you need to establish the correct diagnosis with your primary care practitioner (PCP) before you begin your therapy. Do not try to start therapy before doing this. If your "PCP" does not give an accurate diagnosis (WITH NEURO-MECHANISM GENERATING THE PAIN), then ask for a referral to a specialist. If your PCP does not facilitate this for you, you know what to do at that point...

Secret Number 3: The most common cause of chronic low back pain results from Degenerative Disease.

1) Chronic Low Back Pain from Degenerative Disease

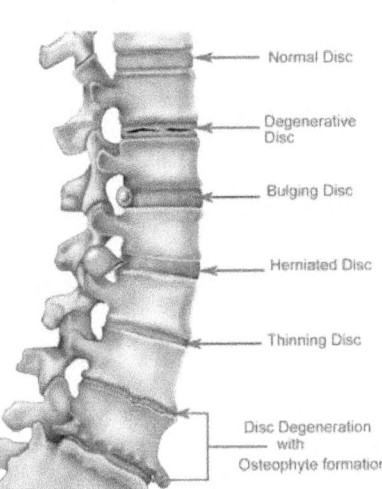

SPINE CONDITIONS

Normal Disc

Degenerative Disc

Bulging Disc

Herniated Disc

Thinning Disc

Disc Degeneration with Osteophyte formation

This degeneration can occur in the joints and discs of the back. When it occurs in the discs it is called Degenerative Disc Disease (DDD). In DDD the "padding" (called discs) between the bones of your spine (called vertebrae) wear out. In that sense, everyone can expect to develop DDD...if they live long enough. Just like a pillow eventually loses its fullness over time, so does every human being's vertebral discs. Perhaps this is not as much "a disease" as it is the normal result of the "wear and tear" that a human body experiences through life.

There **are** certain people who **have** a genetic tendency to develop this earlier in their life than expected. Sometimes you will see entire families with "early" DDD. There is also a greater chance to "wear out" earlier if you smoke, are overweight, have done very physical work during your life, or had experienced some unusual trauma (for example, if you were a paratrooper).

There are several ways that chronic pain is generated from DDD. The disc is a structure that has a rim of tough cartilage on the outside (annulus fibrosus) with jelly in the center (nucleus pulposus). As the disc wears out it becomes flatter, the "jelly" dries out, and if it develops cracks in the rim cartilage, it can "leak" the "jelly" from the center (called a herniated disc).

This all adds up to the neighboring structures becoming crowded, compressed, and forming boney overgrowth.

Local nerves can be compressed, the spinal canal can be narrowed, and the bone overgrowth causes facet joint deterioration (little joints on the top and bottom of most vertebrae). Chronic back pain can be generated by all these processes.

There are several very simple lifestyle changes that you can do to slow down the process of degeneration:

- Stop smoking.
- Stay lean.
- Avoid activities that put stress on your lower back.
- If you must work or perform activities that put stress on your back then consider back bracing during the activity.
- When exercising, develop your "core muscles" which will help distribute the stress on your lower back.
- Choose your parents well (just kidding).

Treatment should target the neuro-mechanism generating the pain. You will need an accurate diagnosis to start with. That will require a thorough history and physical, an MRI of the lumbar spine with contrast, and referral to a specialist that is familiar with DDD (i.e. an Orthopedic Surgeon, Neurosurgeon, Pain Specialist, etc.). Your Primary Care Practitioner (PCP) should be able to coordinate this for you. Under the best of circumstances, a team of people will be drawn together by your PCP.

Practically speaking, your insurance company will place limitations on how extensive your team involvement is.

You will also need to learn what works best to relieve your pain and develop your own treatment regimen. The people who do the best with chronic back pain from the degenerative disease are those who "take charge" of their own therapy.

2) Chronic Low Back Pain from Disc Herniation

DDD can result in actual disc herniation. The most formidable conditions are those that have severe symptoms with a minimum of externally observable findings. Disc herniation is not observable with a physical examination. Nearly every vertebra has a disc. It serves to cushion the movement of each unit and bear the weight of the body. It is made of a very resilient form of cartilage called fibrocartilage. It's the "grizzle" that some of you have eaten in cheap cuts of meat. It is the special taste that is imparted to a Jamaican delicacy called "ox tail" (I am a grafted in Jamaican...my wife was born there).

The fibrocartilage of a disc is arranged in concentric rings called the annulus fibrosus. It is the outer ring of the disc that surrounds a jelly-like material called the nucleus pulposus located in the center of the disc. Together they combine to create a structure that has incredible resilience to twisting (called torsion), bending, compression, and stretching. The disc allows the vertebra to move in multiple ways.

Every tissue of your body is regulated neurologically, is nourished by the vascular-lymphatic-interstitial fluid circulation. Your body is repaired, protected, and sometimes injured by the immune system. It is also subject to other hormonal control mechanisms. The disc is affected by these same processes. The disc has small blood vessels and nerves in and around it. It's "health" is dependent on an ample supply of blood, oxygen, and supportive nutrients. Repetitive injury or disease affects the supply and weakens the structural integrity of the disc. The disc in a sense then "starves" and begins to degenerate.

Secret Number 4: Degeneration of any structure in the human body occurs when the injury caused by destructive forces is not effectively counter-balanced by healing processes.

The conflict between degeneration and regeneration is ongoing. A severe force applied to a healthy disc or a mild force applied to a "starved" disc (degenerated) will cause injury. The symptoms of injury must reach a certain threshold before a person can feel it. If an injury occurs slowly and remains sub-threshold, an injurious process can go on undetected. This is what often happens when a person who had a relatively small trauma (i.e. bending over to pick up a light object) ends up with a herniated disc.

The disc can be injured in a number of ways from a bulge in the annulus (stretching of fibers) to a crack in the annular fibers to frank herniation to fragmentation of the disc. When the disc annular fibers are still intact but stretched asymmetrically, a "bulge" can develop. In a bulging disc, the center nucleus pulposus is still contained by the annulus fibrosus. The disc structure has become deformed but still retains structural organization.

If the outer rim of annulus fibrosis fibers separates, then the nucleus pulposus may flow out of the center and compress structures outside the disc (i.e. such as spinal nerve compression). This is called disc herniation. Spinal nerve compression can give the classic burning pain radiating down a leg. If the separation of the annular fibers swings closed the "jelly" will remain trapped outside the disc and require invasive therapies. If the separation remains open then intensive, non-invasive therapies may be successful to facilitate healing by drawing the "jelly" back into the center of the disc (traction can do this).

Secret Number 5: An MRI does not make the diagnosis of disc herniation all the time.

Even an MRI can miss disc herniation. The strength of the electromagnetic field used in performing the MRI is proportional to its sensitivity in detecting abnormalities. This is measured in Tesla units. I have had cases where the MRI missed a disc herniation that was discovered at the time of surgery. An earlier generation MRI had been used for the spinal evaluation. The "tighter" the anatomy of the area being studied the greater the need for a higher Tesla MRI.

When the extrusion of the center of the disc is forceful or the disc has degenerated extensively, fragments of the extruded material can break off and be forced outside the disc perimeter. The fragments can migrate and cause obstruction of spinal fluid or compression of remote structures away from the immediate vicinity of the original herniation. Fragmentation requires surgical removal and cannot be treated conservatively. In most cases, an open surgical procedure will be necessary to remove the fragments.

3) Chronic Low Back Pain from Spinal Stenosis

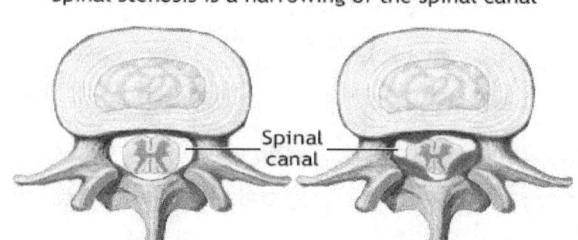

Spinal stenosis is a narrowing of the spinal canal

Spinal canal

Normal   Stenosis

Degeneration can also cause a narrowing of the spinal canal called Spinal Stenosis. In the interior of your spine is a canal called the spinal canal. It is a "boney tube" that runs from your neck to your lower back. It is the home for your spinal cord and spinal nerves. The spinal canal provides protection for your spinal cord (a very fragile structure indeed). Each segment of your spine has the spinal canal within it. As the spine bends so does the canal and your spinal cord.

Any structure that "pinches into" the canal will potentially cause narrowing or "stenosis" (the medical term for narrowing). So you can see that bone overgrowth, disc bulging, tumors, blood, etc. can all cause stenosis. To make matters more complicated, some people are born with a congenitally small spinal canal. In people born with a congenitally small spinal canal, it takes much less damage to narrow the canal and cause symptoms. So goes the old adage, "choose your parents well." The mechanisms for the pain in spinal stenosis (stenosis is narrowing) are many.

Here is a brief summary of how the pain is neuro-generated in Spinal Stenosis:

-Compression of the spinal cord: Nerves do not appreciate being squeezed, cut, torn, frozen, burned, "starved" (deprived of blood or oxygen), poisoned, or stretched. The spinal cord is like a cable with thousands of wires in it. Compression "kinks" the wires.

-Stretch of the spinal cord: As the spinal canal narrows the spinal cord is "tethered" and stretched.

-Ischemia of the spinal cord: Though a rare complication of spinal stenosis, it is possible to reduce blood flow to the spinal cord as the structural damage pinches blood vessels.

-Associated inflammation and degeneration: The muscles, ligaments, tendons, discs, and boney elements of the spine are all close neighbors whose damage can narrow the spinal canal.

The symptoms of Lumbar Spinal Stenosis are mostly what you would expect: low back pain, radiating leg pain, numbness in the legs and feet, and weakness of the legs. However, there are *2 symptoms that are more predictive of lumbar spinal stenosis than other causes of low back pain:*

a) Spinal Claudication (claudication is impairment in walking): This is a curious finding that when people walk they get an increase in their low back pain. If they stop walking, the pain will diminish. This must be differentiated from vascular claudication of the legs (what you would see if the arterial blood flow to the legs was reduced).

b) "Shopping Cart" Claudication: You have probably seen this when you are at the supermarket...people pushing their carts by leaning on them bent at the waist. This is a position of comfort for people with spinal stenosis.

The physical examination will show the usual muscle spasm in the lower back (a general finding in people with back pain), reduced strength in the legs, reduced range of motion of the lumbar spine, and pain when the lumbar spine is forcefully palpated (or touched).

Secret Number 6: There is no single symptom, physical finding, or diagnostic study that diagnoses spinal stenosis.

The diagnosis of lumbar spinal stenosis requires a thorough history and physical by a licensed primary care practitioner. There is no definitive symptom, physical finding, or even test that makes the diagnosis. It is the entire picture of the person that makes the diagnosis. CT Scanning and MRI scanning can diagnose causes for spinal canal narrowing, but there are many cases missed by these tests. The symptoms may be more important than the diagnostic testing.

4) Chronic Back Pain from Scoliosis

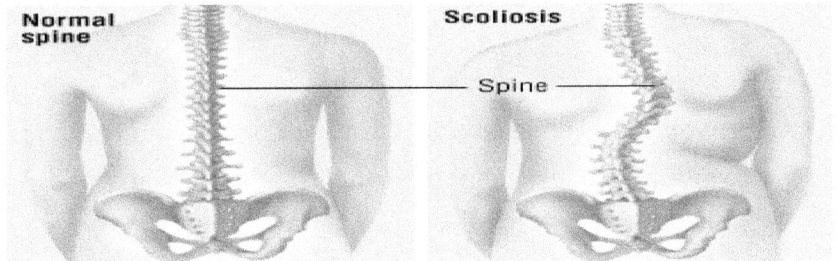

Scoliosis is a deformity of the spine that causes an abnormal lateral curve in the spine. It can occur anywhere along the spine and result in multiple curves. The most common form of scoliosis is Idiopathic (we used to say during our training that an idiopathic disorder has an "idiot physician and a pathetic patient"). This form of scoliosis is genetic in origin (clusters in families). Other causes of scoliosis can be Congenital (present at birth), Neuromuscular (as in cerebral palsy), and Degenerative (such as from an illness or injury).

Generally, scoliosis is more common in females. It is often first identified in children when their mother notices that one shoulder is lower than the other or their clothes are not fitting correctly. These days most physicians screen children for scoliosis so that it is not missed when they are regularly followed. However, growth occurs beyond the pediatric years such that late developing scoliosis can be missed. Identifying scoliosis during the growth years lends itself to be treated by bracing. Later diagnosis (after the growth years) limits the non-invasive options for real treatment.

Most pediatric scoliosis comes without symptoms such that if there is the complaint of back pain an alternate cause for the pain should be investigated. Adult scoliosis more commonly causes back pain, shortness of breath, chest wall pain, and fatigue.

Essentially, scoliosis causes the spine and attached structures to bend, rotate, compress, and apply tension to their attachments. This causes an inefficient movement of the spine with accelerated "wear and tear" (degeneration). The degeneration causes the joints, discs, ligaments, tendons, and muscles of the back to become inflamed. At times, scar tissue can form in the spinal canal as well as in the attached structures. Severe spinal curves can also compress the normal inflation of the lungs (inability to inflate). The process of gas exchange in the alveoli of the lung is affected causing shortness of breath.

The pain of scoliosis is due to the accelerated spinal degeneration that can occur. The tension on nerves, ligaments, tendons, and muscles also generates pain. The curving of the spine causes an enhanced tension and wear of the attached structures (this is particularly true of the facet joints and discs). Finally, chronic inflammation can occur that causes scar tissue in the spinal canal and associated structures. This can masquerade as a herniated disc or a facet syndrome.

Secret Number 7: Calculation of the Cobb Angle is important for determining the actual degree of scoliosis curve. It is also used to guide the type of therapy that may be recommended.

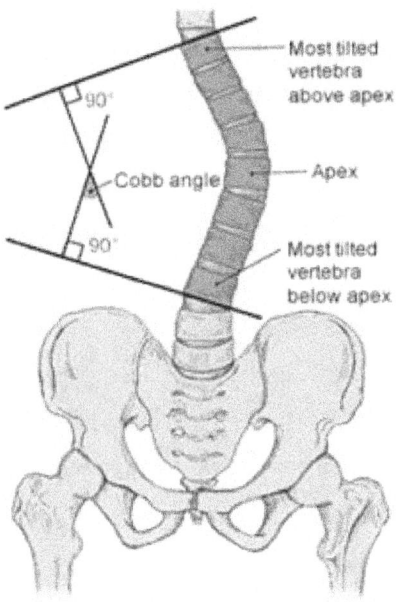

The most important non-surgical treatment for scoliosis is **bracing**. This was first introduced in 1946 and was called the Milwaukee Brace. *Bracing is most effective in young people who have less than a 40-degree Cobb angle scoliosis and at least 2 years of remaining growth.* Adults can also benefit from spinal bracing but will not be able to normalize the curve. Other forms of therapy (chiropractic, massage, injections, ultrasound, etc.) give relief of symptoms but do not reverse the curvature of the spine. They would be expected to give temporary relief at best.

The best therapy for scoliosis is the therapy that will correct, to the greatest degree, the spinal curve. Any other therapy is purely symptomatic and does not address correcting the structural abnormality of the spine. When the Cobb angle exceeds 40 degrees, the person has failed on bracing therapy, or symptoms are worsening the choice for surgery becomes the most effective alternative. The best approach to this form of therapy is to seek the advice of an orthopedic surgeon who has dedicated his practice to corrective spinal surgery for scoliosis.

The surgery for spinal scoliosis can be one of the most extensive of all surgical procedures. The rehabilitation after surgery may take many months. However, the result can be a correction of the spinal curve such that symptoms and progressive deterioration of the spine is minimized. A perfect spinal correction is unusual.

Therapies for Degenerative Disease of the Spine

There are numerous therapies that can be employed in degenerative disease of the back. I like to conceptualize the treatment into non-invasive and invasive therapies:

A) **Non-invasive Therapies:**

- Exercises
- Physical Therapy
- Chiropractic/Osteopathic Spinal Manipulative Therapy
- Acupuncture
- Ultrasound
- Magnetic
- Bracing
- Cold Laser Therapy
- High Density Electrical Field Therapy
- Traction
- Cold Packs/Hot Packs/Substances that heat, cool, or irritate the skin
- Transcutaneous Medicines
- Transcutaneous Electrical Neural Stimulation
- Massage Therapy
- Hypnosis
- Cognitive Psychotherapy
- Prescription Medicines
- Nutraceuticals

None of the listed therapies can remove disc fragments. The mechanisms of healing for the non-invasive therapies is reduction of pain (usually through neuro-mediated mechanisms), increase disc nutrient supply, decrease disc degeneration, reduce inflammation, and realignment of the spine.

B) Invasive Therapies:

- Epidural Injections
- Facet Injections
- Trigger Point Injections
- Micro-discectomy
- Fiberscopic Discectomy
- Intra-spinal Laser Surgery
- Open Discectomy
- Open Laminectomy
- Open Laminectomy with fusion and internal fixation
- Open Discectomy with prosthetic disc replacement
- Corrective Open Surgery For Scoliosis (usually with extensive internal metal fixation)

I will discuss in more detail the multiple therapies used in pain management in a later section of this book. As you can well see all chronic pain of the back does not have the same mechanism for causing the pain. Addressing the exact neuro-mechanism for generating the pain is the essential ingredient for designing the right therapy program and subsequently obtaining relief. You will hear this mantra over and over throughout this book.

II. Chronic Neck Pain Secrets

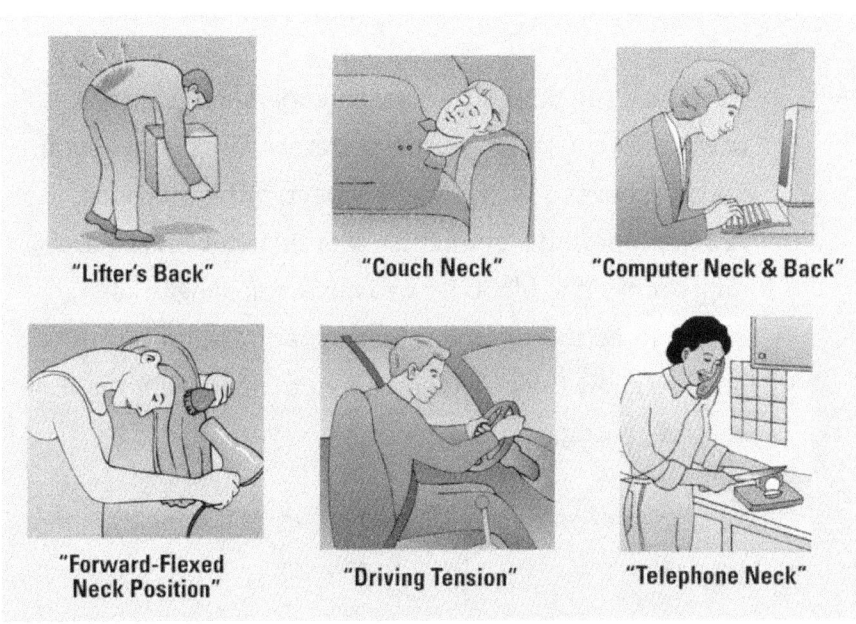

"Lifter's Back"   "Couch Neck"   "Computer Neck & Back"

"Forward-Flexed Neck Position"   "Driving Tension"   "Telephone Neck"

Chronic neck pain (pain continuously for three months or more) is one of the leading causes of disability in the U.S. It is very difficult to "rest the neck" as even lying on your back requires a measure of neck muscle contraction to stabilize your head. This can affect how well you sleep, affect your healing rate, and affect your next day's performance. It has been wisely said, "The next day begins the night before."

Secret Number 1: Chronic neck pain is usually due to one or more of 3 different mechanisms: 1) a muscular problem and/or 2) a skeletal problem and/or 3) a neural (nerve) problem.

Neck pain can be basically broken down into three categories: muscular causes, skeletal causes, and neural (nerve) causes. As you might expect, different causes require different treatments. Muscular causes require improvement in blood flow to hasten healing. Skeletal causes need to have the spine aligned. Neural causes need to allow the peripheral nerve to heal and normalize central neurogenic pain generation.

Secret Number 2: Securing an accurate diagnosis makes the treatments very straightforward.

The best way to treat chronic neck pain is to first know the neuro-mechanism for the pain. This will require a proper evaluation by your medical health practitioner. After you know the mechanism, you can begin the proper method to treat the pain. Many people never learn just what the mechanism for their pain is and never initiate the proper therapy.

One final word on chronic neck pain...it will take time to achieve sustained relief. You may need to apply your specific therapy for six weeks or more. Remember you didn't develop your chronic pain overnight (otherwise it would be acute pain) so you cannot realistically expect it to get better overnight.

In a later section of this book I will review many of the therapies available for chronic pain. The therapies of the neck are very similar to the low back (see the previous chapter for a listing).

III. Chronic Headache Pain Secrets

TMJ

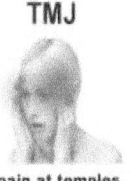

pain at temples,
ahead of ears

Sinus

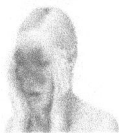

pain at
cheekbones,
above eyes

Cluster

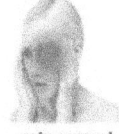

pain around
one eye

Tension

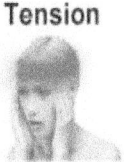

pain "squeezing"
around crown
of head

Neck

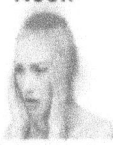

pain in back
of head,
top of neck

Migraine

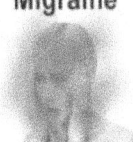

throbbing pain,
nausea, vision
changes, sensory
sensitivity

Mary (her name has been changed) was referred to me as a last resort..."Doctor, I have some type of a headache nearly every day of my life. I have seen Neurologists, Chiropractors, Physical Therapists, Natural Healing Practitioners, etc... None of what they suggested worked. Is there nothing that can be done for me?"

I had heard this story many times before. "Mary, I have reviewed all the records you sent me. You have had a very extensive workup. I think you have Chronic Daily Headache Syndrome and I am going to do my best to get you some relief," I said trying to generate some hope for her.

Forty-five million Americans suffer from chronic recurring headaches. There are 150 different diagnostic headache categories. Headache is one of the most challenging pain syndromes that face physicians today. *The Chronic Daily Headache Syndrome (CDHS) is defined as a recurring headache of unknown cause that occurs at least 15 days of the month over three successive months.* There is no identifiable cause after a proper work-up.

Secret Number 1: In CDHS a headache may not fit any classical description of one type of a headache.

In CDHS, there may be characteristics of multiple different types of headaches in one person. It may also change from episode to episode (which can be very unnerving to both Doctor and person alike). It used to be taught that migraine headaches were vascular in origin where the blood vessels first narrow and then reflexively engorge with blood causing pain from stretching of the blood vessels. Tension headaches were taught in medical school to be the result of a contraction of the muscles of the head and neck. This puts tension on the scalp which causes pain. Sinus headaches occurred when the sinuses "filled up" with mucous and caused pain by pressure. We didn't know what the mechanism of cluster headaches was.

Today we understand that the mechanisms of headache generation are very complicated. In fact, there are often overlapping mechanisms causing the pain in any given headache sufferer. This made the usual, orderly, step-care approach to headache therapy more confusing. Most PCPs today still use a step-care approach to headaches. I take a pragmatic approach and individualize the therapy guided by the symptoms, as best as possible.

Secret Number 2: Causes of chronic headaches that must be treated surgically are identified first.

In the chronic headache syndrome, a person will usually have seen a multitude of Doctors and tried many different therapies. Here is one pragmatic (practical) approach:

- *First make sure that a thorough history, physical, and diagnostic workup has been done.* There should have been a Neurologist's consult and an MRI of the brain (with contrast). Surgically remediable causes for chronic headaches should be ruled out first.

- *Secondly, review all the therapies that "have not worked" as there may have been a breakdown in how the therapies were prescribed or taken.* You don't want to necessarily exclude a therapy that was not correctly administered.

- *Thirdly, begin therapies that will relieve pain immediately and simultaneously begin more long term, slower to work therapies.* This will give hope and relief.

- *Fourthly, aim to transition over to therapies that can be taken long term without adverse consequences.* You may end up on opiate therapy at first (before the slower to work medications "kick in"). You can be weaned from your opiate therapy as the other therapies begin to work. It is important to remember that long-term opiate therapy may be necessary.

In my practice, I was always able to construct a therapeutic regimen that achieved relief of a chronic headache. It often took several visits to find the right combination of therapies to achieve this. If your Doctor is persistent, you will eventually find the combination that works for you.

IV. Chronic Joint Pain Secrets

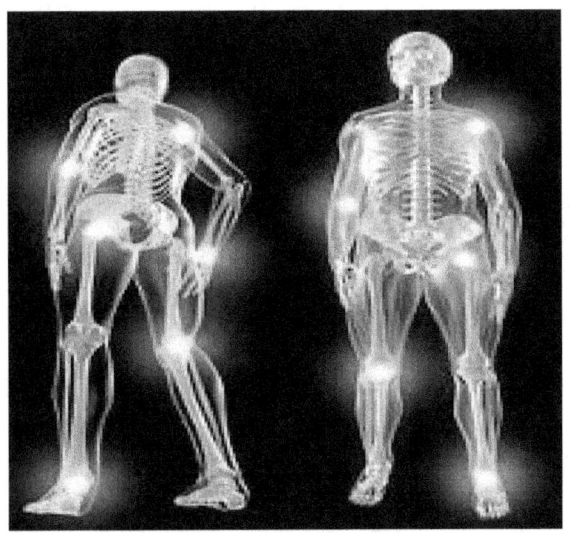

Secret Number 1: The pattern of joint swelling and pain gives clues as to its mechanism.

The presence of swelling ("tumor"), redness ("rubor"), elevated joint temperature ("calor"), and pain ("dolor") lead the Doctor to be able to discern what may be causing a patient's condition. I am going to discuss several patterns of pain and swelling to help you discern the cause of your pain syndrome. Many times the cause can be identified by history alone, before a physical exam and diagnostic testing is performed.

The joints that we will be discussing are all called synovial joints (there are other types of joints too). Synovial joints are specialized joints that contain synovial cartilage. Synovial cartilage is the very "slippery" surface that the major joints of the body move on. Synovial cartilage decreases friction in joints. It looks "purple" to the naked eye. Under the microscope, the cartilage is manufactured by cells called chondrocytes. These cells are embedded in the "pavement" of the joint surface or "matrix." The matrix is spread over the surfaces of bones that rub against each other (called joints).

In a healthy joint, the cartilage matrix is manufactured as quickly as it is worn down. In this way, the joint remains very low friction and painless. In a diseased joint, the replenishment of the matrix is hampered. Sometimes by direct injury, or by infection, or by loss of cartilage, or by an autoimmune inflammatory process (like Rheumatoid Arthritis).

Secret Number 2: The history, physical, and needle aspiration of the affected joint are the starting point evaluation of any joint swelling.

Single Joint Swelling and Pain

Single joint swelling and pain are usually due to a crystal deposition form of arthritis (such as Gout), a direct trauma of some sort, Osteoarthritis, or infection. Single joint infection will usually be due to direct inoculation of infection (such as a puncture wound or skin infection that has penetrated into the joint). You may resist having a needle inserted into a joint that is already painful and swollen. I understand your reticence but, for the most accurate diagnosis, it is necessary.

A sensitive clinician will spray an anesthetic onto the skin before needle puncture (this will diminish the pain but not completely remove the pain of the needle stick). A needle that is at least #18 gauge will be necessary for larger joints as the fluid can be so thick that it cannot be removed with a smaller gauge needle. Once the fluid is removed it can be sent to a reference lab for culture, white blood cell count, and crystal analysis. Be sure that the practitioner who removes the fluid knows what type of tubes to have it transported in. It is ok to ask, "How will the fluid be sent to the lab?"

Interim treatment with an anti-inflammatory such as Motrin will begin to help with the pain and swelling. Depending on the findings of the fluid, the therapy can be further intensified in the following 24-48 hours. The risk of infection is higher if the joint has been previously punctured and if systemic signs of infection are present (fever, chills, etc.). If these signs are present, your practitioner may order an antibiotic too. In some cases you may need to be hospitalized if the infection has become systemic (you will feel like to have the "flu").

Pain and Swelling in Multiple Joints

When pain and swelling occur in multiple joints, it implies a systemic or whole body cause. Usually, this will be due to an autoimmune process (such as Rheumatoid Arthritis) or systemic infection. Systemic infection will be accompanied by fever and chills. The process is similar to single joint management in that a sample of joint fluid needs to be taken from the easiest joint to needle. If systemic signs are present, your practitioner may want to hospitalize you for intravenous antibiotic therapy. It is safer to be aggressive when systemic signs are present as the infection may be in the bloodstream (a more serious cause of joint swelling).

Swelling in a Single Joint without Pain

The cause for this presentation is usually direct trauma of a repetitive type. Over stressing a joint with smaller, painless trauma (such as kneeling) can result in swelling without pain. The singularity of joint findings implies the direct trauma. In some cases, there is no recollection of injury. Management would be the same as before, the joint fluid needs to be examined (it needs to be punctured with a needle).

Swelling in Multiple Joints without Pain

This presentation implies a systemic process that is not arthritic in nature. The most common cause for this presentation is cardiovascular disease. Fluid retention can present this way (such as with Congestive Heart Failure and Kidney Failure). A thorough evaluation by your primary care practitioner will be necessary looking for systemic disease.

Chronic Pain of the Hands

The prevalence of persistent hand and wrist pain ranges from 3% to 26% of the general population. This would mean that upwards of 80 million Americans suffer from persistent hand or wrist pain. Certain occupations and lifestyles can place a person at risk for developing this syndrome (where the hands are used to squeeze repetitively).

The hand is a compact structure of musculo-skeletal anatomy. The majority of grasping and fine finger movement of the hand is powered by forearm muscles located some distance from the hand. The motor power is connected through a complex array of cables called tendons.

The movement of this cable network results in the generation of friction. The friction is minimized by sliding the tendons through well-lubricated coverings called tendon sheaths. Any distortion of the tendon or covering changes the frictional coefficient and can cause pain. The blood and nerve supply to the hand also comes from the forearm into the hand through the wrist. There is an anatomical narrowing at the wrist through which the blood and nerves must pass. Any distortion of the compact narrowing at the wrist can affect the blood and nerve supply to the hand. The central nervous system directs the function of the hand. The amount of neurons assigned to this task is considerable given the complexity of the movements of the hand. Central and peripheral nervous system disease can severely affect the function of the hand (even in the absence of any direct hand abnormality).

Secret Number 3: Diffuse hand pain can be the result of a local or remote disease.

Proper evaluation of hand pain requires the examining clinician to be well acquainted with the complicated anatomy of the wrist and hand. Understanding this anatomy makes the diagnosis of chronic hand pain well within the scope of most primary care practitioners.

The causes of hand pain can be broken down into 7 basic types:

- Disorders of nerves
- Disorders of blood flow
- Disorders of ligaments
- Disorders of tendons
- Disorders of bones
- Disorders of joints
- Disorders of skin and soft tissue

For the purposes of this section we will be confining our discussion to disorders of joints, tendons, and nerves. The volume of information and potential disorders that can occur with the hand precludes an in-depth discussion of all possibilities.

Joints can be affected by a loss of cartilage (Osteoarthritis), inflammation of the joint (Rheumatoid Arthritis), direct trauma, abnormal tissue growth (such as tumors), abnormal blood supply, and abnormalities of the nervous input to the hand. Tendons are subject to nearly the same risks as joints. Nervous system abnormalities can occur through central and peripheral diseases. At times, the dysfunction may be quite remote to the hand but effects the hand enormously (such as in a nerve injury).

3 Common Causes of Joint Pain of the Hands

1) Osteoarthritis (OA):

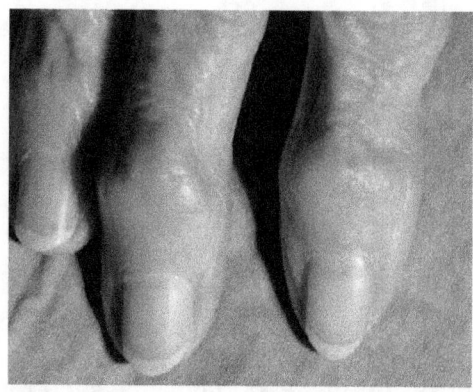

The hand is particularly vulnerable to the "wear and tear" of life. Because of this the most common form of arthritis of the hands is Osteoarthritis. Essentially a wearing away of cartilage in the joints of the hand, OA causes pain and disfigurement of the joints of the fingers. Other joints can be involved too, but the most characteristic changes occur in the last joint of the fingers. These are called Heberden's nodes. People who use their hands for intense activities will develop OA more readily. Though there is a genetic tendency in certain families, joint stress is a major risk factor for OA.

2) Rheumatoid Arthritis (RA):

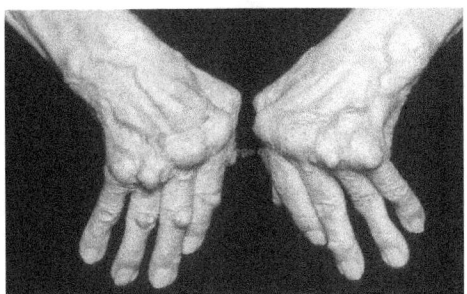

The autoimmune process that occurs in Rheumatoid Arthritis also gives a characteristic appearance to the hand affected by it. The disease process in RA inflames the membrane inside the joint (synovial membrane) causing the release of destructive substances. The destructive substances primarily affect the joint surface but can also affect all the other local structures adjacent to the joint (for instance, tendons and ligaments). The deformity that occurs is also quite characteristic as the hand cycles through many phases of inflammation and healing between acute episodes (see the above picture).

3) Carpal Tunnel Syndrome (CTS):

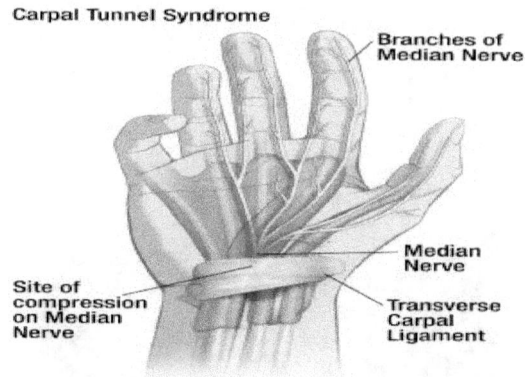

Carpal Tunnel Syndrome

Branches of
Median Nerve

Median
Nerve

Site of
compression
on Median
Nerve

Transverse
Carpal
Ligament

Although not a joint disorder, CTS is a major cause of pain and disability in the hand. The disorder is essentially one of compression of the Median Nerve, which traverses the wrist en route to the hand. Any process that causes narrowing of the aperture through which the Median Nerve traverses, the Carpal Tunnel of the wrist, can cause CTS. The disease process is one of nerve pain and can be very discomforting.

Specific Treatments

The treatment of the three disorders requires general pain treatment as well as having some specific features.

- *Osteoarthritis (OA)*: The primary disease process is one of loss of cartilage on the joint surface, but replacement of the cartilage of finger joints is not possible at this juncture. However, tremendous relief can be achieved with pain medications, anti-inflammatories, and natural pain relievers (such as Turmeric).

- Rheumatoid Arthritis (RA): The inflammation in the autoimmune process of RA is much better treated today than when I was in medical school in 1978. Beginning with the general arthritic treatments (pain medication, anti-inflammatories, etc.) therapy may need to be advanced to an exciting category of medicines called Disease Modifying Agents (DMA).

DMA therapy reduces the actual process of autoimmunity in the person with RA and has resulted in a much more favorable prognosis. This type of therapy is usually administered by a specialist called a Rheumatologist (a specialist in arthritis). Later in this book I review many general treatments for pain which may also be used if you suffer from chronic joint pain of the hands.

- Carpal Tunnel Syndrome: The primary process is compression of the median nerve. All therapies are aimed at decreasing that process. However, if after the usual therapies of splinting, anti-inflammatories and change of wrist use the pain does not remit (usually no longer than 4 weeks), the carpal tunnel will need to be enlarged. This can be done with a non-invasive device called a CTrac or via surgery (see the section on "Carpal Tunnel Therapy Secrets").

Chronic Joint Pain of the Knees

Knee pain is one of the most common reasons people come to their primary care practitioner (PCP). 30% of all orthopedic complaints are related to knee pain. Over 50% of all athletes will complain of knee pain at some point in their lives. Most people underestimate the seriousness of their chronic knee pain. By the time a person presents to their PCP, they are often times past the point where preventive measures could have made a difference. So it is that the USA has the highest rate of knee replacement in the world.

Secret Number 4: The knee is a mechanically "at risk" joint.

You can think of the mechanical disadvantage of the knee this way...2 long poles attached by cords attempting to limit the backward and forward...side to side motion at the ends where the 2 poles meet...that's the knee. When the knee is involved in activity it moves in a multi-planar way (though its major motion is like a "swinging hinge"). In motion, all attachment and cartilage tissues of the knee are stressed. When standing erect the knee rotates slightly, "locks out," and handles its weight load with a minimum of ligament and tendon strain. The knee also has two curious interior structures called menisci (meniscus in the singular). The menisci guide the synovial surfaces of the knee and help decrease the "backward and forward – side to side" motion of the knee. They stabilize the sliding surfaces, disperse friction, and cushion the knee. They are made of fibrocartilage (similar to the substance of the outer ring of a vertebral disc).

Even at bed rest the knee is moving (just ask a friend who has had knee surgery). There is no possible way to eliminate motion of the knee without fusing it. Fusion is a surgical procedure where the femur (upper leg bone) and tibia (lower leg bone) are surgically made into one long pole. Although this may reduce or eliminate knee pain, the additional stress on other adjacent joints often results in secondary dysfunction elsewhere.

The knee is also the most commonly injured large joint of the body. Just watch an athletic contest where there is major body contact and you will see that there is at least one knee injury. It's an "anatomical set-up" that the knee would get injured. Even bracing of the knee gives it little support. Orthopedic studies done on football offensive lineman (the largest people in American-style football) show that a knee brace works by reminding the lineman to reduce the strain on their knees by changing the way they block. It offers little measurable supportive help.

The knee is a "swinging-hinge" mechanism. The actual major motion is in the form of an arc that places stress on different structures within the knee at different phases of its motion. In the standing position, the knee ligaments (which attach one bone to another) and tendons (which attach muscle to bone) are at minimal stress. The major stress standing is compressive and is applied to the cartilage located on the end of the tibia and femur (called synovial cartilage).

As the knee begins to bend, the patellar tendon tension begins to rise first (the patella is the "kneecap"). As motion continues tension in most ligaments and tendons builds to reach maximum stress at the fully bent position (the "squat"). Ligament shearing remains a major mechanism of injury in sports. More recent orthopedic surgical techniques utilizing cadaver ligament and tendon transplants (called allograft transplants), as well as tendon transplants from one part of the body to another (called autograft transplants), have improved recovery from cruciate ligament tears. Ligament looseness (called "laxity"), tendon looseness (also "laxity"), and loss of cartilage of the knee are usual with the aging process. Injury of the knee, at an earlier age, accelerates the aging process of it. If a human being lives long enough, especially one who has had an active, athletic lifestyle, they will develop some category of knee problem.

Causes of Knee Pain

1) Osteoarthritis:

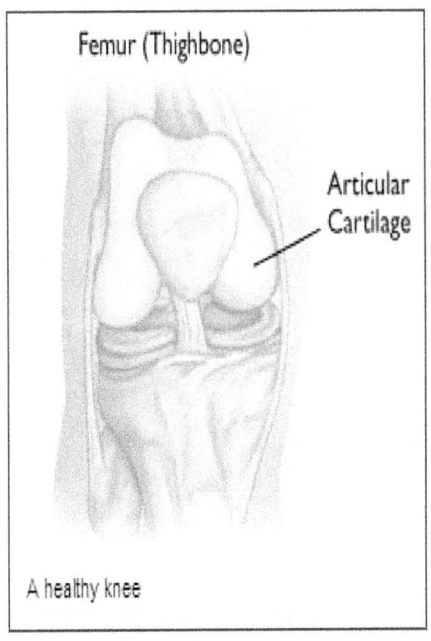
Femur (Thighbone)

Articular Cartilage

A healthy knee

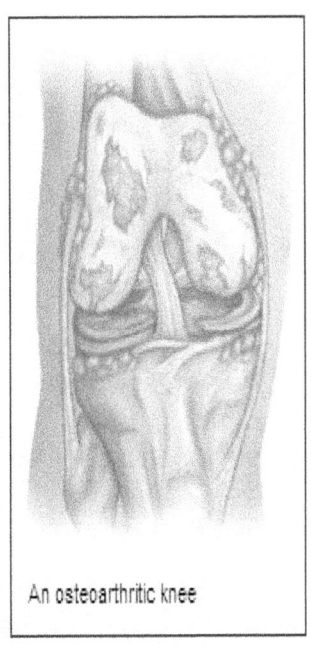
An osteoarthritic knee

By far the most common cause of chronic knee pain, Osteoarthritis (OA) is a process of loss of cartilage from the surface of the femur and tibia. Although partially genetically governed (some families develop this condition at an earlier age), the major mechanism for OA is progressive micro-trauma to the cartilage. This micro-trauma eventually outstrips the healing mechanism of the cartilage. The cartilage then becomes less abundant as the cells that produce it decrease in number. Eventually, pieces of cartilage are lost and "pitting" occurs. This "pitting" is akin to the potholes seen on the streets of major cities after a severe winter. Exposed bone, local inflammation, ligamentous laxity, and reflex muscle fatigue (the body's attempt to stabilize the knee) all contribute to the pain felt in OA of the knee. OA is the most common reason for total knee replacement.

2) Ligament Tears:

As I introduced previously, the knee is at a disadvantage structurally such that tears of ligaments, tendons, and the menisci are common. Ligaments sustain a tear according to the mechanism of the force that is applied. Lateral and medial ligament tearing occurs when a high energy force is applied to the opposite side of the knee. Medial Collateral Ligament tears occur by a lateral force applied and vice versa. Cruciate Ligament tears occur when the applied force is from the front or back of the knee. The Cruciate Ligaments (anterior and posterior) cross in the interior of the knee. As the Anterior Cruciate ligament stabilizes the tibia from going too far anteriorly on the femur, a powerful force directed posteriorly against the femur (from the front) can tear this ligament. This often occurs when the athlete themselves land or pivot awkwardly.

Secret Number 5: The Anterior Cruciate ligament accounts for 90% of the stability of the knee.

An Anterior Cruciate Ligament tear is a common injury in high-velocity contact sports (such as in American-style football). Recovery from this form of injury is difficult. Usually, an orthopedic surgical repair is needed with a tendon transplant. Even with surgery, the rehabilitation from an Anterior Cruciate ligament tear is 1 or 2 years. The good news is that, post repair and rehab, the recovered function is quite good. Many professional athletes have recovered and returned to active status.

Chronic pain after a partial Anterior Cruciate ligament tear can occur if the resultant knee remains loose after healing (and there is no surgical repair). The laxity causes excess motion which injures the menisci and synovial cartilage further. This is called Chronic ACL Deficiency.

3) Meniscal Tears:

Secret Number 6: Tears of a meniscus are often unstable and heal slowly.

As previously eluded to, the Menisci are two fibrocartilage discs that cushion and guide the surfaces of the tibia and femur. The injuries to the menisci occur when a severe shearing or compressive force is applied. As the menisci age, the fibrocartilage becomes less flexible and sustains micro-trauma. As the blood supply to this structure is not robust, healing occurs slowly and is easily outpaced with repetitive micro-trauma. Tearing of the menisci can occur horizontally, vertically, or on an angle. It can also be complete or incomplete. The result can be an unstable tear or a flap. Unstable tears or flaps require very slow and progressive rehabilitation. In many cases, the removal of the involved meniscus is required for relief of pain.

The removal of a meniscus destabilizes a knee further which accelerates the development of Osteoarthritis of the knee. The decision to remove or not remove the meniscus is best advised by an experienced orthopedic surgeon.

Chronic Joint Pain of the Elbow

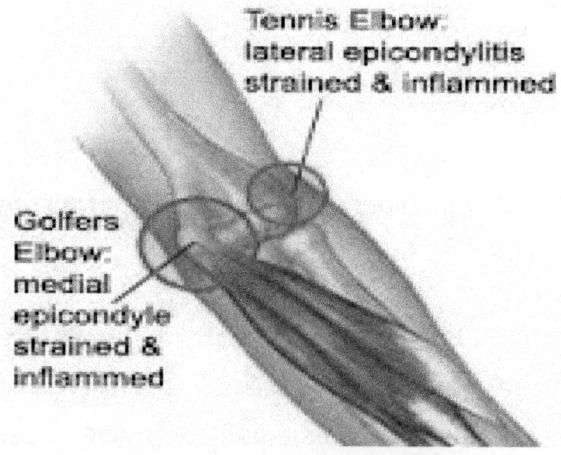

The elbow is a joint that is at some degree of mechanical disadvantage (though not as profoundly as the knee). Chronic pain of the elbow is usually caused by a disuse injury. A disuse injury is one in which the elbow is repeatedly exposed to incremental trauma. Incremental trauma is where the bones, ligaments, and tendons are exposed to small traumatic stresses that cause micro-tears and micro-fractures. These will usually not be visible on plain x-rays of the elbow. They may also not be very obvious on MRI or CT scanning of the elbow. I will be discussing the 3 most common causes of chronic elbow pain. As the elbow joint surface is a synovial joint surface, it is susceptible to the autoimmune diseases (for instance, Rheumatoid Arthritis). The autoimmune diseases of the elbow will not be a focus of this chapter.

The elbow joint has 3 bones in it. The upper portion of the joint is made of the end of the humerus (the upper arm bone), the head of the radius (which rotates on its long axis so that the palm of the hand can rotate a full 180 degrees or more), and the ulna which forms a u-shaped hook onto the end of the humerus. This makes the elbow a rotating hinge joint. On the ends of the humerus, radius, and ulna is synovial cartilage that allows for the low friction movement of the elbow joint (the same type of cartilage on the boney surfaces of the knee). The cartilage thickness is less than on the weight bearing joint surfaces (such as the knee).

Functionally, the humeral-ulnar joint operates with a hinge like mechanism. The radial-humeral joint allows the radius to rotate around the ulna so that the palm can face up or down at will. Both of these joints make up the elbow. The elbow joint is actually 2 joints in one. Important nerves and blood vessels course on the outside and inside of the elbow, generally sparing the middle where the joint motion is occurring. The arteries, veins, nerves, and lymphatics of the elbow are not well visualized on conventional x-rays, MRI, or CT scanning of the elbow. Dislocations, fractures, and crush injuries of the elbow are often complicated by disruption of these poorly visualized structures and require specialized radiographic testing to evaluate (such as an arteriogram or venogram). Elbow disruption of this type will not be covered in this section.

Wherever skin slides over a boney prominence (like a "sharp" angle of a bone) there resides a curious soft tissue structure called a bursa. The bursa functions to allow the skin to move over a joint without having a hole worn through the skin. It is a "pillow" of soft tissue that is normally not seen on physical exam or x-ray. The elbow has a very important bursa just under the skin at the "point" of the elbow.

3 Causes of Chronic Elbow Pain

1) Tennis Elbow (TE):

Tennis elbow (TE) is a disuse injury that can occur any time the elbow in repeatedly rotated outward (a "backhand" stroke in tennis). It can also occur when the hand in repeatedly used in a forced grip action (such as using scissors). Given the mechanism of injury, one can predict which sports and occupations are at risk of developing the syndrome. Tennis, sheet metal workers (due to using sheet metal scissors), seamstresses, etc. can all develop this syndrome.

The pain of TE can be quite severe. It is usually located on the outside of the elbow laterally. Palpation on the side of the elbow usually yields a painful response from the person with TE. There is often swelling and redness in the area too. Plain x-rays are usually normal. The actual problem is the occurrence of micro-tears of the tendons and ligaments attached to the lateral epicondyle (the boney nob where there is pain on applying pressure). The medical term for TE is lateral epicondylitis.

2) Golfer's Elbow (GE):

Golfer's elbow (GE) is a disuse injury that can occur any time the elbow is repeatedly rotated inward (a "forehand" stroke in tennis). As this is the major elbow motion in golf, the syndrome has been named GE. Given the mechanism of injury, one can predict which sports and occupations are at risk of developing the syndrome. Golf, baseball, and occupations that require heavy use of a screwdriver can all cause GE.

The pain of GE can also be severe. It is located on the inside of the elbow medially. Palpation on the medial inside of the elbow causes a painful response from the person with GE. There is often swelling and redness in the area. Plain x-rays are usually normal. As in TE, GE occurs as a result of micro-tears of the ligaments and tendons attached. In this case, the attachment site is the medial epicondyle (the boney nob medially on the elbow where pain occurs with pressure applied). The medical term for GE is medial epicondylitis.

3) Olecranon Bursitis (OB):

The olecranon is the boney tip of the elbow. Olecranon Bursitis is a swelling of the bursa that is positioned just below the skin on the tip of the elbow. OB can occur by direct irritation (direct trauma) or by irritation from an underlying disease process (such as Rheumatoid Arthritis). Bursitis pain can be as severe as inflammatory arthritis. The appearance of OB is classic with a swollen, painful "sack" of fluid over the tip of the elbow. When the bursa is irritated, it produces more fluid than it can reabsorb and accumulation occurs

Secret Number 7: Lateral and Medial Epicondylitis are caused by micro-tears of the ligaments and tendons located in their respective areas.

The treatments for the above conditions are very similar with a few noteworthy variations. All 3 disorders may benefit from the following:

- *Joint Rest:* naturally, an injured joint needs to heal so discontinuing the activity that caused the swelling just makes sense. In some cases, the activity may not be able to be discontinued due to the essential nature of the activity (you may need to use the joint to stay employed).
- *Ice/Heat:* the general rule for this would be ice for 24-48 hours. After the acute phase of swelling then heat. In the case of chronic pain and swelling, heat applied every 2 - 4 hours for 20 or 30 minutes may be helpful by increasing blood flow and removal of tissue inflammatory mediators.
- *Anti-inflammatory Medications:* over the counter medications are usually dosed at the lowest effective dose. Prescription doses may be necessary. If ice/heat/rest do not resolve the pain,

then an evaluation by your primary care
practitioner would be in order.

- *Epicondylitis Strap:* by placing a constriction band
  on the forearm, in front of the elbow, the tendon
  and ligament strain is minimized (the physics of
  how the elbow works). This type of banding often
  yields immediate results and can also be used as a
  preventative if the joint cannot be rested.
- *Transcutaneous Electrical Nerve Stimulation
  (TENS):* by stimulating the muscles and nerves
  around the elbow, blood flow increases with
  reduction in inflammatory mediators. This will
  reduce chronic elbow pain.
- *Bursal Drainage:* this would have to be done by a
  trained medical practitioner. Afterward, the elbow
  is usually encircled with a constriction wrap to
  decrease fluid re-accumulation.
- *Epicondyle injection:* the judicious injection with a
  local anesthetic and steroid can often give
  immediate relief of GE or TE. This would be
  administered by a trained health care practitioner.

If the above treatments are ineffective (most people
would get relief with the above), a referral to a specialist
will need to be coordinated by your primary care
practitioner. A further discussion of treatments follows
later in this book.

V. Menstrual Pain Secrets

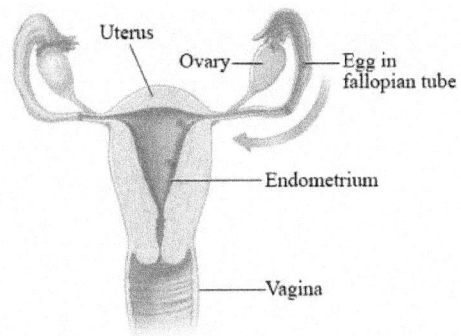

When does a woman with an established pattern of painful periods have to worry? I used to dread the possibility of missing a life-threatening cause of a woman's abdominal pain mistaking it for menstrual pain. I retired from medicine before such a thing ever happened...but I vividly remember the dread.

Even as a trained physician there are real perceptual differences between male and female physicians. I cannot recall a detailed discussion with any female colleagues about their menses. It is part of the female mystique. Male physicians can be at a disadvantage in this area. This is a problem since most physicians are still males.

Secret Number 1: Women have a normal connection from the contaminated outside to the sterile interior of their abdomen.

To complicate matters further, the causes of painful periods are numerous. How can a woman with chronically painful periods discern if a deeper problem is occurring? Unlike men, women have a direct connection to the sterile interior of their abdomen...it is called the female reproductive tract. The introitus of the vagina (entry opening) leads through the vagina to the cervix...then the uterus...through the fallopian tubes...and finally into the sterile peritoneal cavity. Men have no similar conduit from the contaminated outside to the sterile inside.

Also, women hemorrhage internally every month...this is called ovulation (the blood loss is small but real). The egg is released into the sterile peritoneal cavity and "caught" by the end of the Fallopian tube (FT). The egg then traverses down the FT to be confronted by sperm for conception or, in the absence of sperm, proceeds to the uterus to be expelled with the lining of the uterus in what is called a "period" (external hemorrhage). This second hemorrhage in the menstrual cycle can result in quite a bit of blood loss. But, what is often forgotten of the process is the amount of inflammation that accompanies a "normal" period. Inflammation is the process by which the body protects and heals itself. Medicines that reduce inflammation too much can delay or even prevent healing. Inflammation not only occurs in a local area (such as in injury...the ovulation of an egg from an ovary, for instance) but also has a systemic response. Menstruation results in inflammation. Though it is a normal female process, in some cases, the inflammation can be too much. Symptoms remote from the place of inflammation (the uterus) can occur as well as in the uterus. When this happens the usual symptoms of menstruation are accompanied by additional discomfort (joint pain, nausea, behavioral changes, etc.).

Secret Number 2: Women have a normal cycle of hemorrhage and inflammation every month called a menstrual cycle.

In addition to hemorrhage and inflammation, there is a menagerie of hormonal fluctuations occurring with a woman's menstrual cycle. These fluctuations affect nearly every major organ system of a woman's body. The results are a diverse array of symptoms that range from effects upon the nervous system to the gastro-intestinal system. It can be difficult to separate these symptoms from the symptoms caused by independent and unrelated illnesses.

Hemorrhage, inflammation, and hormonal fluctuations can occur with other syndromes. How could one tell the difference between symptoms of the menses alone from overlap with other illnesses?

To begin to discern the symptoms of the usual menstrual cycle from a separate underlying illness, ask the following 7 "high payoff queries":

#1 *"DO I FEEL DIFFERENT FROM MY PREVIOUS PERIODS? "*

Although the nature and severity of a woman's menstruation can vary greatly from woman to woman, each woman will usually establish an individual "pattern" for their cycle. Associated with their pattern will be a set of symptoms that are fairly stable over time. If there is a sudden change in the "pattern" that may be indicative of a change in the physiology of what is going on. There may be a new underlying process occurring.

#2 *"DO I LOOK DIFFERENT FROM MY PREVIOUS PERIODS?"*

I knew a Doctor (she was a world famous forensic pathologist) who felt fine but woke up one morning with yellow eyes while having her period. She felt no different but noticed jaundice (yellowing of the skin and eyes) when putting her make-up on in the morning. Later that same day she presented herself as a case to the medical students she was teaching (she did so without telling them it was her) ...they nailed the diagnosis...painless jaundice…pancreatic cancer until proven otherwise. She died from pancreatic cancer that same year.

#3 "DO MY FRIENDS AND FAMILY ASK ME IF SOMETHING IS GOING ON?"

Our friends and family can often notice subtle changes in us (especially if they haven't seen us for some time). It is possible for new, subtle changes to occur so gradually that the person will miss it. The common saying, "I know myself better than anyone else" is not always true. A curious defense mechanism called "denial" disrupts that axiom.

#4 "DO I HAVE NEW OR DIFFERENT SYMPTOMS FROM PREVIOUS PERIODS?"

Perhaps the easiest question to answer is whether there are new symptoms. Every woman establishes a pattern of their menses. Even if the pattern is "no pattern," the sudden emergence of a new, consistent symptom is evidence of a change in physiology and will be recognized. The symptoms in the menstrual cycle are connected biochemically. Whatever a woman is feeling is a reflection of what is happening physiologically. The feelings disclose the invisible metabolic processes that are mediating her cycle.

#5 *"ARE THE SYMPTOMS OF MY PERIOD THE SAME BUT MORE EXTREME?"*

Sometimes the symptoms don't change but the intensity does. This too discloses a change in biochemical balance. In medical practice, I knew that if a menstruating woman's periods were unchanged, even if there was concern about an underlying illness, the woman could be reasonably reassured that she would be ok. I used a menstruating woman's cycle as a "health barometer" to guide me in looking for hidden disease.

#6 *"AM I EXPERIENCING AN UNEXPLAINED WEIGHT LOSS OR WEIGHT GAIN?"*

The loss of weight without cause (and sometimes weight gain) is a serious finding. I cannot remember any time in nearly 27 years of medical practice that weight loss without cause was a spurious finding that didn't reveal a serious underlying problem. That being said, it did not usually mean that the underlying cause was of a terminal nature. Usually, it was something correctable. In my practice, it was usually the presence of undiagnosed Diabetes Mellitus.

*#7 "WAS MY LAST COMPLETE GYNECOLOGICAL EXAM
OVER A YEAR AGO?"*

There have been several revisions as to the recommended frequency of pelvic examination for women. In my opinion, after nearly 27 years of practice, I never observed any "missed diagnoses" when menstruating women who were sexually active had yearly pelvic exams. A full pelvic exam is a bimanual exam (the Doctor examines the vagina with their hand – by feeling), a vaginal exam (the doctor looks into the vagina with a speculum), and a rectal exam. If all three have not been done, it is not a complete exam, in my opinion.

Secret Number 3: The "7 High Payoff Queries" for menstrual pain may reveal the presence of underlying illness. Answering "yes" to any single question is an indication to have a thorough evaluation by a primary care provider.

I have tried to give some guidance as to determining whether a menstruating woman with painful periods needs to worry about other disease processes that could be lurking unbeknownst to her. The guidelines given above will help you to know when you need to seek medical attention for unexplained symptoms. If you do not ignore these guidelines, you can be confident that a hidden illness, related to your menses, will not be missed.

This information is not intended to be medical advice or replace the thorough history and physical performed by a qualified medical practitioner.

VI. Chronic Abdominal Pain Secrets

Conditions Associated with Abdominal Pain

Right	Center	Left
Gallstones Cholecystitis Stomach ulcer Duodenal ulcer Hepatitis	Heartburn/indigestion Hiatal hernia Epigastric hernia Stomach ulcer Duodenal ulcer Hepatitis	Functional dyspepsia Gastritis Stomach ulcer Pancreatitis

Kidney stones
Kidney infection
Inflammatory
  bowel disease
Constipation
	Umbilical hernia
	Early appendicitis
	Stomach ulcer
	Inflammatory
	  bowel disease
	Pancreatitis
		Kidney stones
		Kidney infection
		Inflammatory
		  bowel disease
		Constipation

Appendicitis
Inflammatory bowel
  disease
Constipation
Pelvic pain (Gyne)
	Bladder infection
	Prostatitis
	Diverticulitis
	Inflammatory
	  bowel disease
	Inguinal hernia
	  (groin pain)
	Pelvic pain (Gyne)
		Constipation
		Irritable bowel syndrome
		Inflammatory
		  bowel disease
		Pelvic pain (Gyne)
		Inguinal hernia
		  (groin pain)

A REAL CASE

Marion and her husband (her name has been changed) were sitting patiently in the examining room when the I walked in. "Hello Doctor", Marion began, "I was referred to you by Pastor Focht, who told us if you couldn't figure out what was wrong with me no one could (I winced as I heard those words). Ever since I had my Hysterectomy I have had a searing pain in my vagina. I had the surgery because of the pain but it didn't help. I am unable to be intimate with my husband. Doc, my life has become unbearable. Every Doctor I have seen tells me to see a Psychiatrist. I never had psychiatric problems before...why do they think I need to see one now?"

Marion has what would be termed "Chronic Pelvic Pain Syndrome in Women". About 15% of all women in the U.S. suffer from this malady. Only a third of women seek medical care for this chronic pain syndrome (of which less than half ever receive a definitive diagnosis). Marion was understandably upset as she queried me. The diagnosis of CPP in women is complicated. Let me put into perspective the difficulties in coming to a specific diagnosis of this condition:

- The first major challenge is that women have pain, hemorrhage internally, and generally feel less well on a monthly basis...this is called menstruation. The process is actually a monthly inflammatory process with hemorrhage.

- The second major challenge is that many women will develop a growth that expands their uterus 800% or more, have a radical fluctuation in body chemistry, and end the process with a traumatic event to their pelvis...this is called pregnancy with a vaginal delivery.

- A final challenge (there are probably more) is that women have a conduit from the outside to the inside that has a tendency to "hide stuff" …this is called the normal Female Reproductive Tract.

It is no wonder that women have chronic pelvic pain. It's a set-up, of sorts. In the usual course of events, women are regularly "traumatized" by their normal anatomy and physiology. The list of possible causes for chronic pelvic pain in women is enormous. Before a woman can be said to have this syndrome, the pain must be present for six months or more (a little longer than the usual three months for chronic pain in other areas of the body).

Secret Number 1: Chronic Pelvic Pain Syndrome in women is not assigned until no other cause for the pain can be discovered after a proper workup. The pain has to have existed for 6 months or longer (this is a little longer than the usual 3 month criteria for chronic pain).

A good history and physical is a starting point for any diagnostic workup. In this case, it was essential to have a very careful history taken with an emphasis on symptom fluctuations associated with menstruation. Even though Marion had many previous evaluations performed by very competent health care practitioners, I proceeded as if I was the first. **A thorough pelvic examination must be performed by an experienced Doctor (with the emphasis** on "experienced" in performing pelvic exams). Marion had already had two thorough pelvic examinations by very competent Doctors. I next proceeded with a methodical evaluation of the consultations and technical studies that had already been performed on Marion to try and secure a diagnosis.

Secret Number 2: The difficulty with human beings is that the anatomy of the pelvis is "tight" and "shielded" by the pelvic bones. The pelvic organs are in very close association in the pelvis. This decreases the sensitivity of the diagnostic studies that are used to evaluate the pelvis.

There is no single test that completely looks at the pelvis...not even a CT scan. The supervising clinician must be aware of the limitations of each diagnostic study that is employed in the search for a diagnosis. This is the area where I found the most variation in practice. Many Doctors have not learned to think critically and methodically consider the diagnostic possibilities.

Secret Number 3: In a diagnostic work-up the supervising physician must understand the limitations of any given study. This is called "critical thinking" and it is crucial for difficult to diagnose disorders.

"I don't want to live if I can't get some relief," was Marion's attitude after having her pain for so long. In her case, she previously had a workup that was very adequate.

Unfortunately, it did not reveal any cause for her pain. When an adequate work-up has not yielded any specific findings, the cause for the pain may be neurogenic or psychiatric in origin.

Human disease does not occur in a vacuum. There are patterns that will emerge when a person is repeatedly examined. Dr. Charles Mayo (of the Mayo Clinic) once re-examined a patient every week, for months, before he was able to see a pattern of symptoms emerge in order to make a diagnosis. I performed a thorough history and physical on Marion.

In Marion's case a pragmatic approach was taken:

1) Her pain was treated aggressively and immediately. She was given a regimen of opiates (a sure fire way to get some pain relief quickly).

2) A second medication that could reduce the nerve impulses of pain (called Lyrica) was started. I will be discussing this very effective medicine in my section on treatment later in this book.

3) A third medication was also begun (to restore neurotransmitter levels to normal) ... a low dose anti-depressant that "recycles" both norepinephrine and serotonin (called Cymbalta). This too will be discussed in a separate section.

The opiate pain meds gave her immediate relief (and hope) while the other medications would take weeks to work.

Many doctors would have just begun the Lyrica and Cymbalta because of the risk of addiction to the opiate medications and potential drug interactions. It is not more righteous to leave a patient in pain because of an unwarranted fear of addiction. It is impossible to treat chronic pain without risk...no matter what is chosen as therapy. Many Doctors would argue otherwise.

On multiple re-visits, Marion's medications required adjustment. She was open and honest about how she was taking her opiate medications (the only way a Doctor can guard you against major side effects). She could not tolerate the Cymbalta side effects so it was discontinued.

In about a year, her pain began to diminish. She was weaned down on her chronic dosing of opiates and remains on just an as needed dose. On her last visit to my office it went something like this:

"Doctor, my pain has gotten as low as a "3" at times. If you hadn't given me the relief I needed when I first met you... I think I would have taken my own life. What would I have done without you?" Her husband sat next to her and wept with joy and relief. Not every patient that presented to my office had such a favorable outcome. However, I cannot recall a time where I was unable to establish some relief for every patient that needed it. Relief for the patient is often a matter of persistence on the part of the Doctor.

CONSIDER ANOTHER CASE OF VAGUE ABDOMINAL PAIN:

Bill (his name has been changed) was pacing in the exam room when I came in. "I am sorry Doc, but I need to go to the bathroom. Do you want a urine sample? I have been like this for over a year." I handed Bill a urine cup to check for infection. A dipstick analysis showed no signs of any abnormality in the urine. Bill's problem was likely chronic.

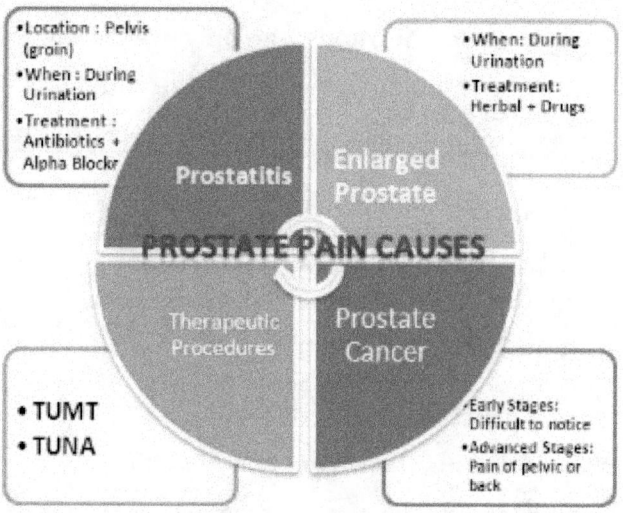

Chronic Pelvic Pain Syndrome (CPPS) in men is defined as pelvic or perineal pain (pain behind the testicles) for three months or more that is not due to a urinary tract infection.

The old term for this was "prostatodynia" or painful prostate. In the U.S.A., CPPS is the most common reason for men 50 years-old and over to see a urologist.

As it turned out, Bill had previously had an extensive workup by an excellent local urologist and was told that "his prostate was fine." He had been given some medicine by the urologist but couldn't remember the name of it... "it didn't work anyways," according to Bill. He told me that when he sits down it hurts behind his testicles (that's why he was pacing when I entered the exam room). He feels like he has to urinate all the time, but when he goes, there is just a small amount of urine. There is no real burning when he urinates...he just has the pain behind his testicles "all the time." "My last Doctor told me it was all in my head," Bill complained. His primary care physician had referred him to a psychiatrist. Bill has the usual non-specific symptoms of CPPS in men. He did notice the pain seems to get worse after he ejaculates (but it hasn't stopped him from having sex). He is a truck driver by occupation.

Secret Number 4: CPPS in men requires 3 months of chronic pain and a negative diagnostic workup. This is a little different from what is required for women.

There are several key considerations when working up a man with CPPS:

1) A thorough workup by an urologist is essential. If this has already been done, have a copy of the results of all the tests e-mailed to your Doctor's office. You may be surprised when you find out that certain key studies had never been done.

2) There are no definitive historical facts, physical findings, or diagnostic studies to diagnose CPPS in men. The diagnosis of CPPS is essentially to rule out other causes for the symptoms a man is complaining about. Since the most common cause would usually be a prostate abnormality, diseases of the prostate remain a consideration in nearly all cases of CPPS.

3) Recent research has suggested that even negative cultures of the prostatic fluid, prostate biopsy tissue, and urine does not exclude the possibility of a prostate infection. Some forms of bacteria require specialized testing to detect them.

4) There is even recent evidence that in CPPS the prostate can become injured by a previous infection and give way to symptoms that masquerade as an infection.

5) The absence of "objective" findings on physical exam or diagnostic testing does not necessarily infer a psychiatric reason for the symptoms.

Remember…a thorough History and Physical, as well as a consultation with a urologist is essential in the evaluation of CPPS in men.

The mainstay of therapy in CPPS is a class of medications called Alpha-Adrenergic Blockers. They work by relaxing the smooth muscle in vital areas in the male Genito-urinary tract (one of the mechanisms for chronic pelvic pain in men). The names are Hytrin, Cardura, and Flomax. Each has benefits and limitations.

In CPPS, a trial of antibiotics is often attempted (the duration of which may be more than a month). Theoretically, CPPS is a non-infectious disorder. However, given the limitations to perform specialized testing (cost, availability, etc.), a one to two-month trial of antibiotics is usually attempted.

Bill was started on an alpha-adrenergic blocker with relief of his symptoms within 24 hours. His pain and urinary urgency improved and he had minimal side effects from the medication. On his last office visit with me he delightfully stated, "Doc, you're a life saver. I didn't tell you before, I guess I was embarrassed, but I was having trouble being intimate with my girlfriend. This new medicine has changed everything." A relatively simple answer to a problem that had plagued Bill for over a year.

Achieving relief for a patient is a very gratifying experience. It is not usually the genius, nor the innate talent, nor the place where the Doctor trained that correlates with the relief of pain for the patient. **The relief of pain for the patient is directly proportional to the persistence of the treating physician to be unrelenting in their pursuit of a diagnosis and treatment for their patient.**

VII. Fibromyalgia Secrets

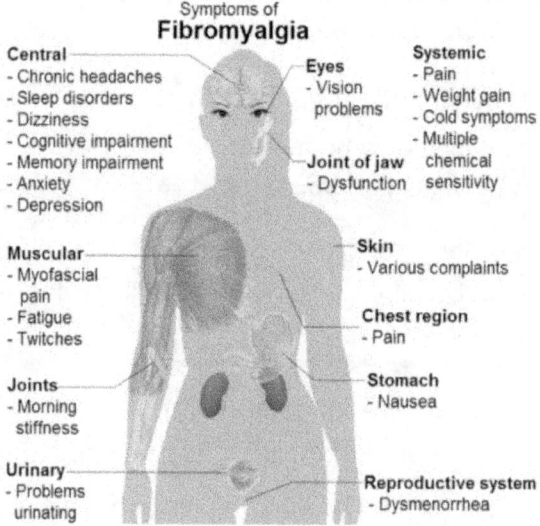

Symptoms of
Fibromyalgia

Central
- Chronic headaches
- Sleep disorders
- Dizziness
- Cognitive impairment
- Memory impairment
- Anxiety
- Depression

Eyes
- Vision problems

Joint of jaw
- Dysfunction

Systemic
- Pain
- Weight gain
- Cold symptoms
- Multiple chemical sensitivity

Muscular
- Myofascial pain
- Fatigue
- Twitches

Skin
- Various complaints

Chest region
- Pain

Joints
- Morning stiffness

Stomach
- Nausea

Urinary
- Problems urinating

Reproductive system
- Dysmenorrhea

A REAL CASE

A young woman and her husband were waiting anxiously in the exam room, "What seems to be troubling you Stella..." I asked her? "I am so uncomfortable Doctor. I ache all over, I have trouble sleeping, I have no energy, and I am depressed. I have been to several primary care physicians who all referred me to a psychiatrist. I am not crazy! I was fine just a few months ago (her husband rolls his eyes) and now I feel like I need to go on disability." I looked at Stella's husband who said, "Doc, we haven't had sex in months...you have got to do something now!"

If this sounds familiar, then you have become acquainted with a common contemporary syndrome called Fibromyalgia. Although Fibromyalgia (FM) has probably been around since the early 1820's (called muscular rheumatism at that time) the syndrome was officially recognized in 1990 by the American College of Rheumatology. Guidelines were published in an attempt to help diagnose this very uncomfortable disorder.

Secret Number 1: There is no specific test that confirms the diagnosis of Fibromyalgia.

FM is characterized by diffuse pain, fatigue out of proportion to physical activity, mental slowing, and difficulty sleeping. FM occurs 7 times more frequently in women than men and tends to cluster in families. There is an association with depression. There is no specific diagnostic study that confirms the diagnosis. It is usually diagnosed after other likely causes have been eliminated.

The location where the abnormality originates is thought to be in the central nervous system. This is because of the diffuse nature of the symptoms in FM and its association with other psychological disorders (depression for one). Dr. Mohammed Yunus, MD has suggested that

FM belongs in the category of a syndrome he calls the "Dysregulation Spectrum Syndrome" (DSS). Essentially DSS is a disruption of the neurotransmitters in the brain with the resultant effect on hormones and nervous function. As the nervous system is connected to every part of the human body, the symptoms of FM are widespread and variable.

Secret Number 2: Fibromyalgia has no specific therapy that works for everyone. The disorder is probably related to a neurotransmitter defect and is unique to each person.

The treatment of FM is non-specific. If you look at the treatments through a "conceptual lens" it would seem that nearly all treatments can be seen to affect the neurotransmitter levels in the human brain. Exercise, massage therapy, diet therapy, and nutraceutical supplements are all aimed at up-regulating neuro-transmitters.

A promising form of treatment (being administered under a doctor's care exclusively) is as structured by Dr. Hinz **at www.neuroreplete.com.** His method utilizes a high dose supplement which is supposed to restore the neurotransmitter balance in the brain. I do want to emphasize that this form of care for FM must be directed by a licensed physician. According to an article written by Dr. Stevan Cordas, the results that Dr. Hinz has had with his regimen have been consistently positive. This is in contrast to the mixed results that most other therapies yield.

As can be imagined, it is really difficult to search and try multiple different treatments while feeling so uncomfortable. A person suffering from this malady must persist in trying multiple different therapies to finally discover what works for them. I have observed that those who do so will eventually discover a regimen that works for them. The key factor is to not give up!

In the therapy section of my book, you will be introduced to many therapies. Their application as a treatment for Fibromyalgia must be individualized to you. You will have to try various combinations of therapies until you find what works for the type of Fibromyalgia you have. Your neurotransmitter disruption may not be the same as others who have the same symptoms.

Secret Number 3: Fibromyalgia is one of the few pain syndromes that is relieved very poorly with opiate therapy. If opiate therapy gives any relief, it is usually very temporary.

Use a practical approach to finding your specific therapy mix. Start with the therapies that you can begin without a prescription and share your findings with your primary care practitioner (PCP). Have your PCP guide you through the process. In Stella's case, I started her on Lyrica and

Cymbalta. The Lyrica has a central and peripheral neural mediated mechanism to decrease pain transmission. The Cymbalta recycles norepinephrine and serotonin. This helped with her mood and pain transmission. I referred her to a Complementary and Alternative Care clinician who added several supplements to augment cellular metabolism. By her third office visit, her symptoms were beginning to improve. I increased her Lyrica and Cymbalta to the maximum allowable doses (see the section on each for a more specific discussion of these prescription medications). In 12 weeks, her symptoms had improved to the point where she was able to engage in graded exercise without provoking a great deal of pain. By six months, her symptoms had improved to the point where I was able to see her every three months.

Stella's improvement is not uncommon. Understanding that the replenishment of neurotransmitters takes time is essential in the treatment of Fibromyalgia. These guidelines are not to be considered medical advice. If you have Fibromyalgia, share this chapter with your PCP and have them supervise your care. There is hope for your pain relief.

Chapter 6 – Secrets of Uncommon Chronic Pain Disorders

I. Complex Regional Pain Syndrome (Reflex Sympathetic Dystrophy) Secrets

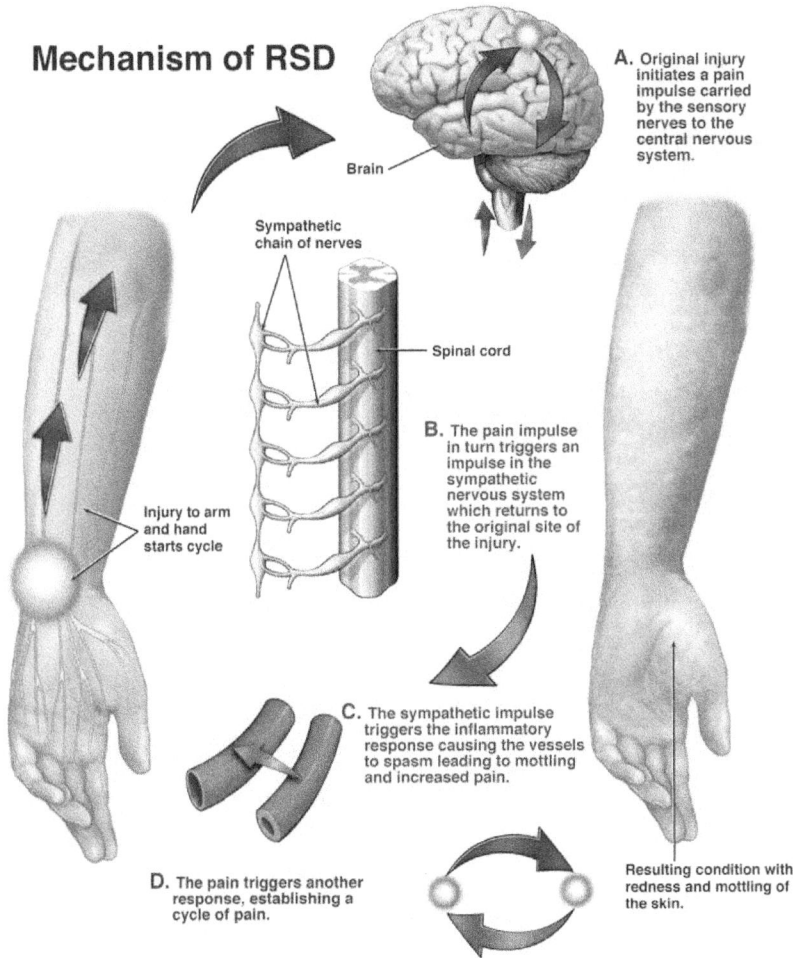

Mechanism of RSD

Brain

Sympathetic chain of nerves

Spinal cord

Injury to arm and hand starts cycle

A. Original injury initiates a pain impulse carried by the sensory nerves to the central nervous system.

B. The pain impulse in turn triggers an impulse in the sympathetic nervous system which returns to the original site of the injury.

C. The sympathetic impulse triggers the inflammatory response causing the vessels to spasm leading to mottling and increased pain.

D. The pain triggers another response, establishing a cycle of pain.

Resulting condition with redness and mottling of the skin.

A REAL CASE

Maria (the patient's name has been changed) was an athletic 20-year-old college student who was on a full athletic scholarship to college for field hockey. While in a "scrum" on the field she was thrown to the ground by an opposing player dislocating her right shoulder (her dominant arm). She was taken to a local Emergency Room (ER) and had her shoulder reduced by the Orthopedic Surgeon on call for the ER. Her relief of pain was nearly immediate and she was placed in a sling and scheduled for follow-up.

Within several hours, her right arm pain restarted but had a burning quality to it. When she saw the Orthopedic Surgeon later that week he told her she probably had stretched the nerves going into her arm when she dislocated her shoulder. He gave her a mild narcotic and reassured her it would get better...it didn't.

Over the next several weeks, the pain became so severe that she stopped her right shoulder rehabilitation exercises. To lightly touch the skin of her right arm caused pain (called allodynia). At the next appointment with the Orthopedic Surgeon he gave her the bad news...she was probably developing a mysterious disorder called Complex Regional Pain Syndrome. He told her that the medical profession was not certain how the pain was generated and that she would have to "learn to live with the pain."

He had rarely seen anyone get relief with any known therapies.

This true story may seem dramatic and rare but it is not. Thousands of people, usually young women in the age group from 20-35 years of age, suffer from the mystery of Complex Regional Pain Syndrome (also called Reflex Sympathetic Dystrophy). **The pain in this syndrome is usually out of proportion to the original injury or what can be seen on physical exam.**

Secret Number 1: CRPS can occur with or without an injury.

The history of CRPS is often associated with an injury of an extremity...but it doesn't have to be. CRPS II is commonly associated with a nerve injury, while CRPS I is not. Patients will often find their treating medical practitioner reluctant to make the diagnosis (they may even be told they have a psychiatric condition). Patients often find themselves searching for a medical practitioner who will help them obtain relief from the intense pain (practitioners are reluctant to give potent pain medications to patients who do not have a positive objective test for their pain).

Secret Number 2: The physical findings of CRPS are non-specific.

The physical findings of CRPS are:

- Temperature changes of the affected extremity (cool or warm).

- Skin Changes of the affected extremity (redness and/or swelling).

- Allodynia of the affected extremity (pain when lightly touching the skin).

- Nail changes of the affected extremity (pitting or brittle nails).

- Painful motion of the effected extremity.

- Hair changes of the effected extremity (loss of hair).

- Abnormal sweating of the effected extremity.

Secret Number 3: There are no specific diagnostic studies for CRPS.

The following studies are often performed to rule out other causes for the symptoms:

- Needle Nerve Conduction Study

- Magnetic Resonance Imaging

- Triple Phase Bone Scan

- Neural Scanning (checks for small, unmyelinated C-fiber nerve function)

- Thermography

There are many curious aspects to CRPS. Just why some people will develop the syndrome (there is some family clustering) from the same trauma that most people do not develop the syndrome remains a mystery. There has, as yet, been no consistently identifiable physiologic abnormality in the nervous system that accounts for the development of CRPS. When the medical profession cannot identify the cause of something, it is nearly impossible to structure a reliable treatment regimen for all people afflicted.

More than likely CRPS has multiple causes that result in similar symptoms. CRPS also has a tendency to "cross-over" to the other extremity (that was previously uninjured). This has led Neuroscientists to speculate on a central nervous system cause for CRPS. Furthermore, treatments that affect the central nervous system have shown some promise for pain relief (the medication Lyrica for instance).

There is no one treatment program that works for all cases of CRPS. It would seem to make sense that, if the mechanism generating the pain is of central nervous system origin, the treatments should be aimed at affecting central mechanisms. These would include:

- *Central Acting Medications*: the spectrum of medications is large (from antidepressants to opiates). Lyrica and Cymbalta are medications often used to treat this disorder.

- *Central Acting Nutraceuticals:* you will have to do your own research and a "trial and error" approach.

- *Non-invasive Therapies that effect the Central Nervous System:* Osteopathic Manipulative Therapy, Chiropractic Therapy, TENS unit, Cool Laser Therapy, Massage Therapy, etc.

- *Invasive Therapies that effect the Central Nervous system:* Spinal Cord Stimulator, Ketamine Infusions, etc.

Because the mechanism for CRPS probably varies from person to person (or at least the nervous system location of the mechanism), the mix of treatments that give you relief will vary from that of another person with CRPS. Nevertheless, as you will read over and over in this book, don't give up. You will eventually discover the combination that works for you.

II. Phantom Pain Secrets

Common Types of Phantom Limb Pain

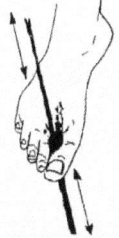

A rope burn sensation between the big and second toe.

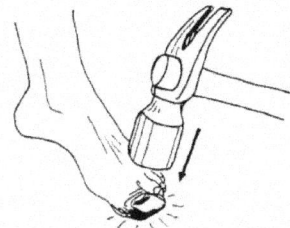

A hammer is smashing the big toe.

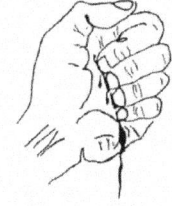

The fist is so tightly clenched that the finger nails are digging into the flesh in the palm of the non-existent hand.

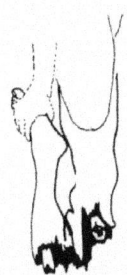

A feeling, for an above-knee amputee, that the fibula and tibia are being broken in half.

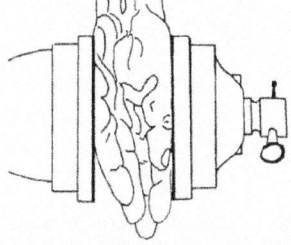

The hand is being crushed in a press.

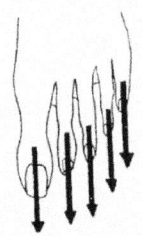

Five toes are being stretched.

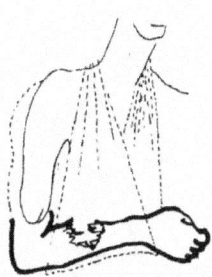

The bones of the non-existent arm are being shattered.

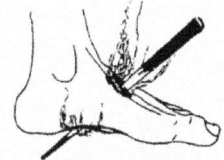

A red-hot poker is being thrust through the foot.

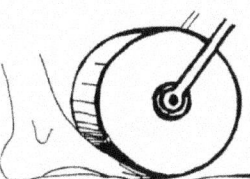

A steam roller is running over the front part of the foot.

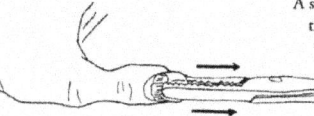

Pliers pulling out nails.

No one grows up thinking they will have a body part removed during their lifetime. Every year 185,000 people in the U.S. have an amputation of one sort or another. Afterward, many will be visited by a phantom and it will be a pain for life. This section will discuss the enigma of Phantom Limb Pain...pain described to be in the region of an amputated body part.

Secret Number 1: Phantom Pain can occur in nearly any region of the body that has had a body part removed.

Most Phantom Pain (PP) occurs in people that have lost a limb. One in every two hundred Americans will have an amputation. The most common causes are a vascular compromise (often due to Diabetes Mellitus) in 54% and trauma in 45%. However, PP does not just occur in limb amputations. Women who have had a Mastectomy, men who have had a Prostatectomy, people with teeth extracted, and even those that have lost an eye may all suffer from PP. Essentially any body part that has been removed can be a "set-up" for PP. People who have PP are often reluctant to disclose it. They sound a bit crazy and realize it. Many are referred for Psychiatric consultation by their Primary Care Practitioner. Fortunately, most amputees do not end up with PP. While 60 to 80% of amputees have phantom sensations shortly after the amputation, most will resolve within six months. The unfortunate few that continue to have PP beyond 6 months often have the syndrome for the rest of their life.

*Secret Number 2: Phantom Pain can manifest with many
different types of sensations.*

The amputee with PP has to not only cope with the
physical, emotional, and financial effects of amputation,
but with PP too. The sensations in PP are not just
restricted to burning pain (see the above diagram). Some
people feel a tightness or squeezing. If their hand is
amputated, they may describe the sensation as a tightly
clenched fist on the amputated side! Tingling, heat, and
cold are also described. Nearly any sensation that could
be detected before the amputation may be experienced in
the amputated body region in PP.

The pain in PP may not be consistent. The general rule is
that the discomfort can be provoked by many different
factors. Stress, anxiety, changes in weather, sexual
activity, light touch, smoking, urination, and even
defecation may all provoke the discomfort. The
provocation may occur despite the stimulus being quite
remote to the amputated body part.

*Secret Number 3: The exact mechanism of Phantom Pain
is unknown.*

The exact physiologic reason that PP occurs is still
uncertain. There appears to be an interaction between the
severed nerve fibers of the amputated body part and the
pain processing area in the brain associated with that body

part. Sometimes the severed nerves are able to generate pain impulses on **their** own. They may, in fact, be over-sensitive once they have healed. This "auto-generator" then interacts with the sensory portion of the brain normally connected to the amputated body part.

The brain also needs regular input of information to function normally. When an amputation occurs, the usual information from that body area is lacking. The associated brain area devoted to the amputated body part becomes "starved" for information and eventually "reassigns" the brain region with a new body part. So it is that blindness can result in exquisite hearing (consider Stevie Wonder or Ray Charles). The tendency to develop PP is higher in people who had a long period of time where the amputated part was malfunctioning before amputation. It is almost like a neurologic "wind-up" occurs. Also, severe traumatic amputations (such as in war) have a higher likelihood of PP. This may be due to emotional "wind-up" related to warfare.

Secret Number 3: The treatment of Phantom Pain varies for each individual.

Up until recently, treatment was fairly ineffective. But, with the advances in our understanding through Neuroscience, a number of very promising therapies have been developed. Here are a few:

- *Biofeedback:* Adaptive control of autonomic functions through learning.

- *Medications:* Anti-depressants, Opiates, Anti-epileptics, and some natural remedies.

- *Acupuncture:* Effects neuro-transmission by cutaneous reflexes.

- *Massage Therapy:* similar to acupuncture

- *Hypnosis:* reduces central pain mediation through distraction called "disattention"

- *Relaxation Training:* causes the release of endorphins (naturally occurring pain-reducing chemicals in the brain).

- *Physical Therapy:* as per relaxation training.

- *Vibration Therapy:* as per relaxation training.

- *Transcutaneous Electrical Nerve Stimulation:* similar mechanism to acupuncture.

- *Local Injections of the stump:* reduces severed nerve irritability in the amputated body part.

- *Spinal Nerve Blocks:* reduces nerve transmission for pain perception.

- *Sympathetic Nerve Blocks*: as per spinal blocks.

- *Spinal Cord and Brain Deep Stimulation:* mixed mechanisms of action in the spinal cord and brain.

- *"Mirror Box" Therapy:* This is one of the most effective forms of treatment for PP. Essentially the mechanism for it is to "trick" the brain into thinking that the amputated part still exists. It is only useful in body parts that can be visualized.

All of the therapies mentioned above have been shown to have some effect on reducing the pain of PP. If you or a loved one suffer from PP, you may need to use a combination of different therapies to achieve the most relief.

THE INFORMATION ON PP IS NOT TO BE CONSTRUED AS MEDICAL ADVICE. YOU MAY NEED TO GO TO A PAIN MANAGEMENT CENTER TO ACHIEVE THE BEST RELIEF OF PP.

III. Multiple Sclerosis Secrets

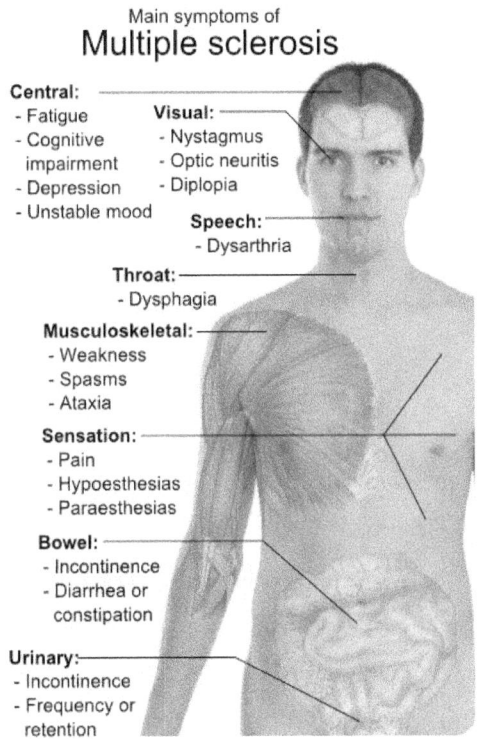

Main symptoms of
Multiple sclerosis

Central:
- Fatigue
- Cognitive
  impairment
- Depression
- Unstable mood

Visual:
- Nystagmus
- Optic neuritis
- Diplopia

Speech:
- Dysarthria

Throat:
- Dysphagia

Musculoskeletal:
- Weakness
- Spasms
- Ataxia

Sensation:
- Pain
- Hypoesthesias
- Paraesthesias

Bowel:
- Incontinence
- Diarrhea or
  constipation

Urinary:
- Incontinence
- Frequency or
  retention

A PERSONAL CASE

Nick is my older brother. He was my protector, mentor, and confidant. He was a man of integrity. He was a real brother. In many ways, we were opposites. I never knew him to lie, cheat, steal, curse, be unfaithful to his wife (he married his childhood sweetheart Nancy whom he fell in love with at 14 y.o.), or dishonor my parents in any way. He served his country in the United States Air Force. He is a man of honor...a rare man. It just didn't seem right when Nick developed Multiple Sclerosis in his third decade of life. I was reminded of all this when he died on Christmas day 2014. He was 65 years-old and had a life of struggle with Multiple Sclerosis. Multiple Sclerosis (MS) is no respecter of persons.

Secret Number 1: The symptoms of Multiple Sclerosis are many and can vary from day to day.

I was in my second year of medical school when Nick was officially diagnosed with Multiple Sclerosis. He had a series of mysterious, painful syndromes...abdominal pain, knee pain, and thigh pain. 50% of patients with MS have chronic pain. Nick's symptoms had become so severe that he could no longer work for General Motors (he had a physically demanding job).

He complained of muscle spasms, muscle twitching, muscle weakness, a loss of balance, difficulty walking, and eventually visual problems (I am sure I am leaving out some of his symptoms). Part of his frustration was not just the persistence of the symptoms...that would have been enough. But, he also used to describe for me the variability of the symptoms. One day's symptom set was different from the next. There was no predicting it.

And then there was that curious problem with taking a hot bath...he found himself unable to get out of the hot water (even though he was able to get in with no trouble). Nick's descriptions were vivid and emotional. They have been etched into my soul.

In the early stages (Nick spent nearly two decades bedridden) you could not tell Nick was ill if you saw him sitting in a chair. It wasn't until he tried to walk that anyone would notice the peculiar way he walked...called a "scissor gait" by medical people. In this type of gait the person cannot relax opposing muscles so they walk hunched over and legs bent continually. It looks similar to people with Cerebral Palsy. MS continued to disrespect him and in a few years Nick became paraplegic (paralyzed from the waist down). He later would become quadriplegic (paralyzed from the neck down) and bedbound. None of the available therapies in the 1970s had any effect on the progression of the disease. He could only experience and chronicle what was happening to him.

Secret Number 2: The symptoms of Multiple Sclerosis are caused by the malfunction of systems that are connected to demyelinated neurons. Neuron demyelination is the mechanism for the disease.

If I may get a little technical for a moment, I would like to explain what the destructive process is in Multiple Sclerosis. You see, nearly any symptom that can be produced by any other disease can be produced by MS. MS is a disease process where the "insulation" of nerves is injured and lost. This is called demyelination. The process is self-consumptive or what is called an autoimmune phenomenon. The body fails to recognize itself as self. The demyelinated nerve cells "short circuit" so that whatever organ they are attached to malfunctions.

The very immune system that is designed to protect us from infection and help us heal in injury plunders the MS patient. Any nerve anywhere in the body can be scourged. So it is that the symptoms can present in an infinite array of patterns. What triggers this to happen is still not completely known. People who live in cold regions tend to have a greater risk of developing MS. This implies some environmental sensitizing agent.

When Nick was stricken with MS, Magnetic Resonance Imaging (MRI) was not yet developed. In fact, CT scanning was still in its adolescence. The Doctors struggled to diagnose Nick's case. Doctors were hesitant to label a patient with MS in 1979. Many other diseases could mimic it. Furthermore, there was little hope for a cure at that time. My generation of physician lived by a credo, "Don't let hope die before the patient." If we couldn't delay the disease, at least we could delay the hopeless diagnosis (rarely a wise thing to do).

Eventually, all other reasonable causes for his symptoms were eliminated and Nick was diagnosed with MS. Today, the diagnosis is more readily established after a thorough History, Physical Examination, and MRI scanning. Fortunately, the necessity for a lumbar puncture ("spinal tap") and special diagnostic studies on the fluid obtained is less necessary these days (a difficult procedure for most people).

Nick spent most of his adult life battling MS. He survived as long as he did because his wife was his dedicated caregiver. She was his Joan of Arc...his protective warrior. Every patient with a chronic illness should have a Nancy. Nancy's life was also plundered. MS didn't respect her life either.

Secret Number 3: Disease Modifying Agents for MS are a promising category of medications that reduce the demyelination of neurons.

Today there is a multitude of medications that modify the aberrant immune function in MS (called DMAMS – Disease Modifying Agents for MS). In the most common type of MS called "Relapsing-Remitting MS" these agents decrease the progression. There still is no absolute cure, but DMAMS give hope. With the present therapies available the unrelenting progression to severe disability can be greatly slowed down. Perhaps Nick's outcome would have been different if he had developed MS today. Ongoing research continues to press for a cure for MS.

Other complicating symptoms are better treated today too (such as pain). The approach to the treatment of pain in MS is similar to the more generic treatment of nerve pain. An extensive listing of pain therapies is discussed later in this book. Nearly any therapy that is effective for nerve pain may be used in the MS patient with chronic pain.

The future for the patient with MS is becoming more hopeful. Cases like Nick's should become less and less common. As for Nick, he watches us from Heaven finally free of Multiple Sclerosis.

IV. Vascular Pain Secrets

SECRETS OF ARTERIAL DISEASE OF THE LEGS

Arterial and Venous Circulation of the Legs

Not all chronic pain of the legs is from arthritis or muscular disease. Some pain can be caused by the blockage of blood vessels in the body. Arterial blockage that happens suddenly is associated with dramatic symptoms. In any location of the body, abrupt blockage of arterial blood flow is catastrophic to the organ system being supplied. Heart attack (called Acute Myocardial Infarction), Stroke (called Cerebrovascular Accident), and blood clot in the lung (called Pulmonary Embolism) are medical emergencies and require emergency attention.

However, a slower more gradual obstruction of arterial blood flow can be subtle in its symptomatic presentation. In other words, the symptoms can be mistaken for other disorders. The dysfunction that results is not as dramatic initially. Chronic pain of the legs can be caused by gradual arterial obstruction of the arteries of the legs.

ARTERIAL DISEASE ANATOMY AND PHYSIOLOGY

The legs require an enormous flow of oxygen-rich blood when exercising. The flow of blood is less at rest and raises dramatically with exercise. Muscle varies in its oxygen requirements depending on whether it is actively contracting or not. At rest, the leg's blood flow requirement is substantially less and can be maintained even though there are severe blockages of the major arteries. The pain of arterial disease of the legs can be evoked by exercise. The same patient may be without any pain at rest.

Secret Number 1: An arterial disease of the legs is usually a gradual process and can cause chronic pain in the legs while walking.

Gradual narrowing of the arteries through atherosclerotic disease is the most common cause of reduction in arterial blood flow. The process is a slow one and may take years to develop. As the flow decreases the vascular system responds by creating collateral arteries that naturally attempt to bypass the blocked areas. Collateralization does not restore the normal flow but is effective in forestalling death of tissue in the legs (until the atherosclerosis is very advanced). The amount of collateralization that occurs is dependent on several factors (such as genetics, gradual onset of the blockages, exercise habits of any given person, etc.).

The development of atherosclerosis is a combination of the forces that push cholesterol into the wall of an artery, the forces that make the wall of the artery "leak" so that cholesterol deposits more easily, and the absolute levels of cholesterol. If you understand these 3 processes that interact to cause the blockages, then you will understand why the risk factors work the way they do.

CAUSES OF ARTERIAL DISEASE

The following are the predominant risk factors in developing atherosclerosis of the lower legs (and elsewhere too):

- Tobacco smoking

- Hypertension

- Diabetes Mellitus

- Hypercholesterolemia

- Genetics

- Obesity

- Autoimmune Diseases

- Sedentary Lifestyles

- Radiation Exposure

- Environmental Toxins

- Chronic Stress States

- Hormonal Imbalance

There may be other risk factors, but this list constitutes the majority of factors that increase the risk of developing atherosclerosis.

Secret Number 2: The risk factors for the development of atherosclerosis of the arteries of the legs are related to blood pressure, cholesterol level, and permeability of the lining of the arteries (allowing them to "leak" cholesterol into the arterial wall).

SYMPTOMS OF ARTERIAL DISEASE

As I have previously stated, leg artery blockage symptoms can be subtle. *The most common symptoms that a person may develop are as follows:*

- Painful cramping in your upper or lower leg muscles with or after activity. This is called Intermittent Claudication. It is usually relieved by a short rest.

- Leg numbness

- Leg weakness

- Coolness of the leg (especially when compared to the other leg).

- Sores on the toe, foot, or leg that will not heal.

- A change in the color of the skin of the leg.

- Slower hair growth on the lower legs (or even hair loss).

- Slow growth of toenails.

- Erectile Dysfunction

- Shiny skin of the legs

- A weak pulse or absent pulse in the legs.

It is also of note that stroke and heart disease are associated with leg artery blockages. It stands to reason that blockages in one area of the body places you at risk for blockages elsewhere.

DIAGNOSIS OF ARTERIAL DISEASE

The history usually reveals one or more risk factors for the development of this disease. After that, pain with leg activity combined with many of the symptoms aforementioned will usually make the diagnosis. Once the diagnosis of leg artery blockage is considered it is easily confirmed. However, the clinical diagnosis itself is not enough to establish a proper therapeutic plan. The next step in establishing a clinical diagnosis from a thorough history and physical is to have Doppler Ultrasound testing of the legs.

The Doppler Ultrasound is a non-invasive, painless way to identify whether there are blockages and to what degree. It will also tell you the location of the blockages so that a complete picture is obtained. It is performed by an Ultrasound technician as an outpatient procedure. A device which emits a dense ultrasonic beam is aimed at the locations of the arteries in the leg. The information is then recorded and evaluated by a physician trained in interpretation of the findings. After that, most people will have a Vascular Surgery consultation for the best treatment plan recommendations.

TREATMENT OF ARTERIAL DISEASE

Secret Number 3: The treatment of atherosclerosis of the arteries of the legs is to prevent further arterial narrowing and relieve severe blockages. Intense reduction of risk factors may result in partial reversal of existing atherosclerosis.

The treatments are based on the severity of symptoms and the findings on the Doppler Ultrasound. Treatment of leg artery blockage symptoms is directed at the causes of atherosclerosis as well as at relieving the blockages. All risk factors that can be reversed should be done so. Smoking must be immediately discontinued, blood pressure controlled, and blood sugar brought to normal.

A referral to a Vascular Surgeon is essential. He/she will perform additional diagnostic testing that measures the actual blood flow reductions, locations of the blockages, and the type of blockage. This will require measurement of blood pressure in your arm and ankle (called the ankle-brachial index or a/b index). The blood flow to your ankle should be equal to or greater than your arm (an index of

1.0 to 1.4). Values below or above the normal range indicate an arterial vascular problem.

Once the blockage has been thoroughly evaluated, the Vascular Surgeon will decide whether intensive medical therapy or surgical procedure is advisable. The underlying concept is to restore adequate blood flow to the involved leg. Most vascular surgeries today involve a procedure called angioplasty. In this procedure, the blocked or narrowed artery is opened with a balloon instrument in the operating room. Because the blockages have a tendency to "spring- back" after the procedure, a device called a stent is often left in place to keep the artery open.

Only the most severe blockages will require an open surgical procedure called vascular bypass.

THERE IS HOPE

Overall, the therapies for arterial blockages are quite good and the outcomes are excellent for people. A return to the painless use of the legs is the norm for most people. For those people who have inoperable, severely advanced disease, control of pain symptoms may be the only alternative. Under such circumstances, the therapies listed later in this book may be all that can be offered.

SECRETS OF VENOUS DISEASE OF THE LEGS

Another very important vascular system of the human body is the venous system. It is a network of thin-walled, muscular tubes called veins. The veins are assigned to carry blood back to the heart so that the oxygen and nutrients that have been removed can be replenished.

The venous system of the legs is arranged into the deep veins, the communicating veins, and the superficial veins. The proper functioning of all is necessary for the effective function of the venous system in the legs.

Secret Number 1: Venous disorders are not caused by atherosclerotic disease (as in arterial disease). Venous disease is caused by trauma to the venous system as a result of increased pressure.

VENOUS ANATOMY

The superficial venous system can often be seen just under the skin surface of the legs. There is a "bluish hue" to the color of the superficial veins due to the blood in the veins having lower oxygen content. The superficial veins collect and return blood from the tissues closer to the surface of the skin and transfer it, through the communicating veins, to the deep venous system. The anatomy of the superficial veins and communicating veins follows a rather loose organizational pattern.

The deep veins of the legs are directly responsible for carrying blood to the large veins in the pelvis and then back to the heart. The deep venous system has a predictable and well organized organizational pattern. These veins are not observable upon surface examination of the skin.

VENOUS PHYSIOLOGY

The main physiology of the veins is to transfer blood back to the heart. This transfer of blood to the heart is called *venous return* (VR).

VR of the legs is powered by three processes:

1) The pumping action of the heart creates a flow that pushes blood through the tubular vascular system.

2) Through a miraculous construction using the principles of physics, the flow pressure on the arterial side is higher than on the venous side such that a pressure gradient "draws" the blood back to the right side of the heart (a "siphon-like" mechanism).

3) The third process is the "pumping action" of the foot and calf muscles to propel the blood in the legs up the tubular network into the pelvis.

Whereas the blood flow from the legs up into the pelvis is against gravity (while in the seated or standing positions) there has to be a mechanism to keep the blood flow from "backing up" in the legs. This is accomplished by valves that normally exist within the venous system. You can think of the valves like the rungs of a ladder, each valve allowing the blood to move from valve to valve (each being separated from each other a short distance). The venous system of the legs is regulated by the nervous and hormonal systems. It is a finely tuned symphony of activity when functioning properly. So what happens when things go awry?

VENOUS PAIN CAUSES

Essentially, pain from the venous system can occur three ways:

- *Stretch:* when the veins are stretched they activate receptors in the walls of the veins that send pain impulses to the spinal cord and up to the brain.
- *Trauma:* direct injury to a vein releases substances that activate pain receptors that send impulses to the spinal cord and up to the brain.
- *Inflammation:* this is a process where the wall of the vein activates the immune system of the body which causes the release of substances that also activate pain receptors that send impulses to the spinal cord and up to the brain.

The two most common causes of venous pain of the legs are the following:

1) Varicose Veins

Varicose veins (VV) are veins that have been stretched out. This usually occurs when the valves of the affected veins are not working properly. When the valves malfunction the pressure inside the vein goes up stretching the vein and causing pain. Previous injury to the vein or simply family genetics are usually the cause.

2) Venous Clots:

A clot is where blood has been activated to congeal and form a plug. The process is normally in a balance as small breaches in the veins and arteries occur quite naturally. The body is forming and dissolving small clots throughout the body all the time. A clot becomes a problem when it restricts the blood from flowing through the vein. This is called thrombophlebitis. Under such circumstances, the pressure inside the vein rises severely injuring the interior of the vein (normally very smooth) and rerouting the flow of blood through alternate pathways. The pain can be quite excruciating.

DIAGNOSIS OF VENOUS PAIN

Varicose Vein (VV) pain is usually quite obvious. The superficial veins of the legs are very apparent with multiple twists and turns. The veins may actually be painful to the touch. The skin can be inflamed that overlies the VV. Occasionally the veins will spontaneously rupture releasing the trapped blood (which is quite dramatic when it happens).

Secret Number 2: Venous obstruction comes from clotting rather than gradual narrowing from atherosclerotic vascular disease (as in the arterial system).

Venous clots are easily diagnosed when they are in the superficial system. As with VV the area is painful and inflamed. Spontaneous rupture is rare, but the pain is usually more severe than with VV alone. If the venous clots occur in the deep system of veins, the diagnosis requires more elaborate testing. As with VV and a superficial clot...pain, redness, and swelling are usually present. Because a more extensive obstruction to blood flow usually occurs with deep venous clotting, the pain and swelling of the leg are usually more severe.   More elaborate testing is required to be able to evaluate how extensive the deep clotting is. Extensive deep clotting increases the risk of all or a portion of the clot to break off. If this happens, the "plug" of clot is rapidly transported through the heart to the lungs. If large enough it can cause sudden death.

The extensive nature of a deep clot is readily identified with a procedure called Venous Duplex Ultrasound. This procedure is easily and rapidly performed by an ultrasound technician. It measures the size of the clot and evaluates for blood flow. Once determined, an accurate estimate of the risk for the clot to break off can be made.

COMPLICATIONS OF VENOUS DISORDERS

The most common and serious complications of venous pain disorders are as follows:

- *Swelling and discoloration of the affected leg:*

Once the veins of the leg have been damaged, there is often a permanent problem with venous drainage. This results in elevated venous and capillary (very small blood vessels) pressures with chronic leakage of fluid, blood cells, and proteins into the tissue. The skin will become "tattooed" with red cell pigment (called hemosiderin) giving the skin a brown color. The tissue will also have an accumulation of fluid called edema. The swelling can often be imprinted with an examining finger (leaving a "dent") for many minutes. It can even become impossible to wear shoes and other foot gear.

- *Ulceration of the skin:*

The tissues that are fluid overloaded are more fragile than normally. Small cracks and punctures will develop into fissures and ulcers. The ability to heal these local areas of injury and infection is reduced due to the reduced blood flow. In severe cases, the ulcers can become quite large and difficult to treat.

- *Recurrent Clot Formation:*

The damage caused by the initial clot can permanently injure the interior of the vein. This causes the likelihood of clot formation to recur due to the reduced and turbulent blood flow.

- *Venous Thromboembolism:*

A devastating complication of venous clotting is the possibility of the clot breaking off and traveling to the heart and lungs. The sudden obstruction of blood flow in the lungs acutely elevates lung pressures which can cause the heart to fibrillate. Death ensues shortly after that.

TREATMENT OF VENOUS DISORDERS

Secret Number 3: Venous disorders are not treated by dilating the vein but by removing the clot and reducing the tendency for the clot to reform.

Axiomatic to most blood flow disorders, the flow of blood through the veins must be restored through various treatment modalities. This is can be done as follows:

1) Reduce tissue fluids and increase venous blood flow:

Leg elevation, compressive stockings, and inflatable pneumatic devices can all reduce tissue fluid and increase venous blood flow. Of course, any ulcers that form need to be directly treated with antibiotics applied to the ulcer or even taken systemically (by mouth or by injection).

2) Reduce the tendency for clot formation:

These types of medicines are called hemorheologic medicines (medicines that affect the coagulation of blood). Aspirin, Heparin, Coumadin, etc. are all agents in this category. Some medicines cannot be taken by mouth and have to be given by injection.

3) Remove clots that are present:

This can be accomplished with medicines that actually dissolve the clot (such as Tissue Plasminogen Activator or TPA) or by surgical removal (where the clot is actually mechanically pulled out of the vein). The clinical urgency dictates how aggressive treatment must be (such as in pulmonary embolism). In many cases, a combination of the above treatments will be used.

THERE IS HOPE

Venous pain of the legs is a very treatable cause of leg pain. The diagnosis is easily established by a licensed medical practitioner. Treatment is very effective when initiated early in the venous injury process. Occasionally there can be no effective direct treatment to the area where the veins are injured or have a clot. Under such circumstances, symptomatic control of the venous pain is all that can be done. The usual generic pain treatments for chronic pain are then utilized. I found in nearly 27 years of medical practice that I was usually able to relieve the venous pain no matter how extensive the venous disease had become.

V. Temporomandibular Joint Dysfunction Secrets

Do you suffer from any of the following?

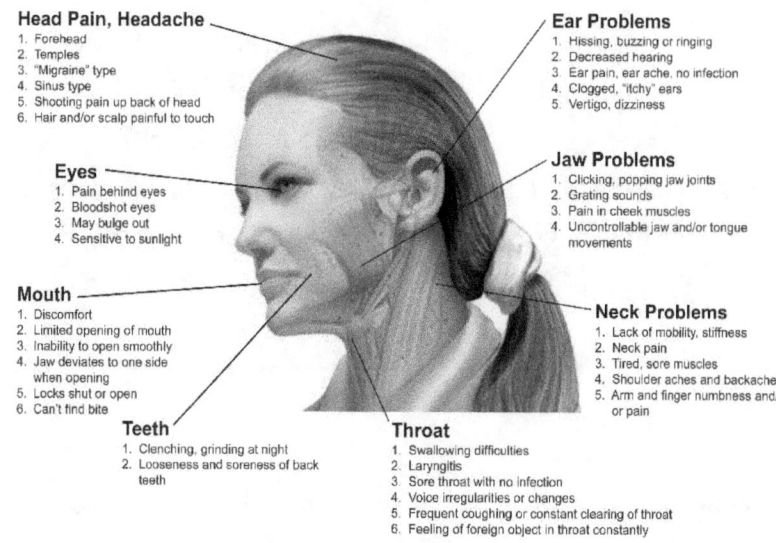

Head Pain, Headache
1. Forehead
2. Temples
3. "Migraine" type
4. Sinus type
5. Shooting pain up back of head
6. Hair and/or scalp painful to touch

Eyes
1. Pain behind eyes
2. Bloodshot eyes
3. May bulge out
4. Sensitive to sunlight

Mouth
1. Discomfort
2. Limited opening of mouth
3. Inability to open smoothly
4. Jaw deviates to one side when opening
5. Locks shut or open
6. Can't find bite

Teeth
1. Clenching, grinding at night
2. Looseness and soreness of back teeth

Ear Problems
1. Hissing, buzzing or ringing
2. Decreased hearing
3. Ear pain, ear ache, no infection
4. Clogged, "itchy" ears
5. Vertigo, dizziness

Jaw Problems
1. Clicking, popping jaw joints
2. Grating sounds
3. Pain in cheek muscles
4. Uncontrollable jaw and/or tongue movements

Neck Problems
1. Lack of mobility, stiffness
2. Neck pain
3. Tired, sore muscles
4. Shoulder aches and backaches
5. Arm and finger numbness and/ or pain

Throat
1. Swallowing difficulties
2. Laryngitis
3. Sore throat with no infection
4. Voice irregularities or changes
5. Frequent coughing or constant clearing of throat
6. Feeling of foreign object in throat constantly

Temporomandibular Joint Syndrome (TMJ) or more accurately Temporomandibular Joint Dysfunction (TMD) is a pain disorder related to the "jaw joint." Pain is not only felt in the joint but can be felt elsewhere on the face. It is more common in women than men, can be permanent or temporary, can occur on either sides of the face (or one side), and occurs most commonly between the ages of 20 to 40 years-old.

Secret Number 1: TMJ can masquerade as other disorders by being associated with neurologic, dental, and other symptoms.

It is characterized by pain in the jaw joint, face, neck, shoulders, and even the ear. The pain is typically made worse by speaking, chewing, or talking. A person with TMJ may notice a clicking in the jaw joint, swelling, tenderness, grinding, or even jaw locking. Symptoms can also be rather misleading with headaches, toothaches, dizziness, hearing problems (such as ringing in the ears called tinnitus), or even upper shoulder pain (see the above diagram). The general cause of TMJ is inflammation of the jaw joint, jaw muscles, jaw muscle tendons, jaw muscle ligaments, or a combination of these structures. At times, the cause is rather mysterious and unidentifiable.

TMJ CAN BE INDUCED BY:

- *Direct injury:* such as a blow to the jaw.

- *Indirect injury:* such as in whiplash.

- *Grinding of Teeth:* such as at night called "bruxism."

- *Nearly any cause of arthritis:* the temporomandibular joint is a sliding synovial hinge joint and is susceptible to disease from Rheumatoid Arthritis and Systemic Lupus Erythematosus (as other joints are).

- *Stress:* causing "clenching" of the teeth

- *Dental Caries:* especially when there is an asymmetrical motion of the jaw joint.

This particular disorder is best diagnosed by a good Dentist. After taking a thorough history, your Dentist will perform an examination of your entire mouth and jaw looking for possible causes for your pain.

TMJ DIAGNOSTICS

There are a few diagnostic studies that your Dentist may perform to confirm the diagnosis of TMJ:

- Facial X-Rays: these will yield what the facial structure is and if there is asymmetry.

- MRI: this study is particularly well suited to evaluate the disc in the center of the jaw joint.

- CT of the face and jaw: this will give a more detailed evaluation of the bone structures.

On occasion, your Dentist may refer you to an Oral and Maxillofacial surgeon (this is not an Ear, Nose, and Throat or ENT surgeon).

Secret Number 2: There is no definitive test for TMJ.

TMJ TREATMENTS

The treatments are usually effective with most people obtaining relief with home remedies:

- NSAIDS: Advil, Motrin, and Aleve (or their equivalents) are usually very effective for pain relief.

- Night Guard: this can be obtained without a prescription and is very effective when regularly used at night. It keeps the jaw slightly open (which rests the joint) and keeps the teeth from grinding at night. A football mouth guard can substitute if a night guard is too expensive.

- Hot/Cold packs to the jaw joint (20 minutes on alternating with 20 minutes off).

- Jaw Stretches: a gentle opening of the mouth with your fingers to stretch the jaw muscles.

- Soft Foods: reduces the stress on the jaw joint.

- Avoidance of extreme movements of the jaw: such as in singing, yelling, or yawning.

- Avoid resting the chin in the hand

- Relaxation Techniques

If these simple modalities do not work then the following therapies can be pursued under the direction of a Dentist or specialist:

- Dental Work

- TENS unit

- Anxiety Medications

- Anti-Depressants

- Ultrasound Therapy to the jaw joint and other painful areas.

- Cold laser treatments

- Radio-frequency treatments

In the event these non-invasive therapies don't work, then the indication for invasive treatment may become necessary:

- Trigger Point injections or direct TMJ injections

- TMJ Arthroscopy: a small scope is put into the TMJ (while under anesthesia) to evaluate and treat the joint.

- Open surgery to the TMJ: this is the final, most aggressive therapy and is reserved for the most severe cases.

Secret Number 3: There is no single definitive treatment for TMJ.

On occasion, you may not discover a "cure" for your TMJ. Under such circumstances, your best alternative is to treat the pain caused by the TMJ realizing you may need to continue the therapy for life. In my practice of Pain Management, I was usually able to help my patients obtain pain relief by blending multiple modalities of treatment.

In some cases, long-term use of opiate pain medications will be necessary.

VI. Spinal Cord Injury Pain Secrets

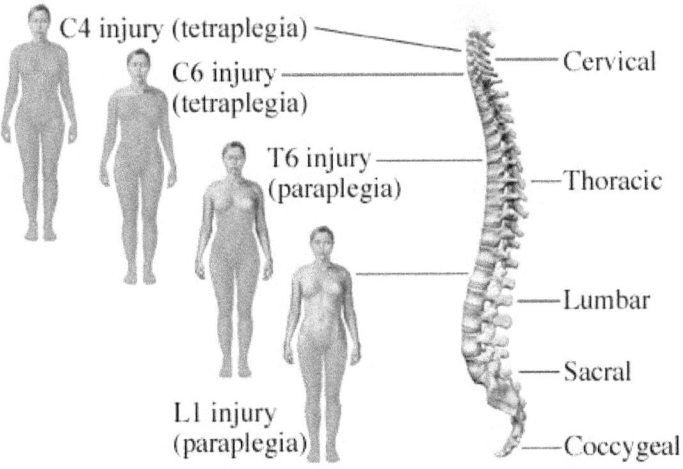

Spinal cord injury (SCI) was usually a lethal event up until World War II. The poor soul that survived was subjected to a world confined to a wheelchair (at best), little social helps (such as graded curbs), and recurrent infections (urinary and pressure sores). The irony of war caused advances to occur that improved the survivability of people with spinal injuries. Improvements in antibiotics, treatment of pressure sores, and advancements in the surgical stabilization of a traumatized spine radically improved survival. The lethal complications of SCI...urinary sepsis, pulmonary embolism, pneumonia, and pressure sore infections have become more manageable. Early interventions for these complications have substantially improved the life expectancy of people with SCI.

SCI STATISTICS

- There are at least 12,000 spinal cord injuries per year in the U.S. (that is, new injuries).

- 250,000 to 450,000 Americans live with the results of a SCI (65% in chronic pain).

- The estimated cost is 9.7 billion dollars per year (I always cringe at cost disclosures).

- The largest proportion of SCI is due to car accidents (followed by falls and violence).

- The average age at injury is 42.6 years (implying decades of supportive care will be needed).

- 80% of SCI patients are men (implying a significant restructuring of family's that have a member with a SCI).

These statistics do not include the war injuries that our brave men and women are suffering defending our liberty against terrorism. Today, improved emergency room care with high dose steroids, spinal protocols, immediate transfer to a neuro-intensive care unit, immediate neurosurgical intervention, and a host of treatment improvements have markedly improved the SCI patient's survival.

What remains a major management issue is spinal cord injury nerve pain. With improved survival in SCI the long-term management of chronic pain remains challenging and frustrating. The rehabilitation of people with SCI and chronic pain is markedly reduced.

The exact mechanism of pain in SCI is still incompletely understood. It would appear that spinal pain after SCI often worsens as healing occurs. People who have had a gunshot SCI seem to be at a greater risk for developing chronic spinal pain.

SCI is divided into Complete and Incomplete spinal cord injuries. The Complete Type results in total malfunction below the level of injury. The Incomplete Type has some residual function below the level of spinal injury (whether it be sensory function, motor function, or both). Curiously, people with the Incomplete Type are at greater risk for developing chronic spinal pain.

POSSIBLE MECHANISMS OF PAIN

The possible mechanisms for chronic spinal pain are as follows:

- Nerve cells make new connections in the brain and spinal cord in response to SCI (called neuroplasticity).

- Nerve cells create new relationships with supportive cells (called Glial cells).

- Nerve cells become more easily excited.

- Nerve cells are less inhibited.

All in all, there are so many changes that occur it is difficult to sort out which ones cause the spinal pain syndrome. Also, there are many people with the identical injury that do not develop spinal pain. You might think that having a SCI would leave a person painless and paralyzed from the level of the spinal cord injury downward. As I said before, about 65% of people can have "pain" above or below the level where the spinal cord is injured.

Secret Number 1: The same spinal injury may give different spinal syndromes in different people.

The central nervous system is affected by many factors. It is the single most reactive organ system of your body to environmental stimuli. That reactivity has a certain amount of pre-programming genetically, but it is not restricted to genetics. It will also change in response to the variations of stimuli from the environment. Imagine if your computer could "rewire" itself in response to the way you used it. It would come with a built-in structure but, within a short time, it could adjust its structure according to the programs you used, or the internet searches you did, or even the way you interacted with it. Well, that's what your central nervous system does. With nearly 100 billion nerve cells in the brain, each with thousands of connections, each changing according to the environmental stimulus...the number and types of connections exceed the number of known stars and planets in the universe (no exaggeration).

 Secret Number 2: There are 9 different pain syndromes that can occur with SCI.

To intelligently treat the pain of SCI, it is subcategorized into nine types. I will briefly describe each and its treatment:

1) *Spinal pain: this is pain that arises from tissue damage of the bones, ligaments, and tendons of the spine.* It is essentially skeletal pain. It responds to many of the treatments that would work for degenerative joint disease. Acetaminophen, anti-inflammatories, and opiates all help this type of pain.

2) *Muscle spasticity pain: this is pain that results from the prolonged contraction of a muscle from denervation.* Though it will respond to the treatments for spinal pain, the most effective treatment is Baclofen. Baclofen is a muscle relaxer that is particularly well suited to treat muscular spasticity caused by nerve damage.

3) Overuse pain: this is pain that occurs in areas that sustain extra "wear and tear" due to the SCI. For instance, the shoulders and wrists are often injured in paraplegics (people with an SCI that results in leg paralysis). The therapies described for spinal pain would be useful for this type of pain.

4) Internal Organ pain: the person with a SCI can have a dysregulation of internal organ function. Because the internal organs receive their "instructions" for function by way of the spinal cord, disruption of the normal function of the spinal cord affects the internal organ function. This can happen even if there is no direct injury to the organ. This is a vague but discomforting syndrome where the person may feel cramping or bloating. There is no treatment. The episodes usually remit on their own.

5) Nerve entrapment pain: SCI patients can develop "pinched nerves" just as any other person. Their description of the pain will depend on the level of their spinal cord injury. The symptoms and treatment would be according to the nerve trapped.

6) Spinal Cord swelling pain (called syringomyelia): in this type of pain the spinal cord has swollen due to a blockage of spinal fluid flow. The patients will usually describe a burning pain. This syndrome develops years after the initial injury. Surgical treatment is the only effective option...the blockage has to be relieved.

7) *Transitional Zone pain: this is a burning sensation that occurs on the border of the skin at the level of the SCI.* It is treated with the medications that relieve other types of nerve pain.

8) *Psychological pain: it goes without saying that depression, anxiety, etc. can be manifested as pain or worsen existing pain.*

9) *Central pain (called the central dysesthesia syndrome):* This is the most difficult of all the pain syndromes associated with SCI. The mechanism for this pain syndrome is poorly understood and treated. The SCI patient will complain of pain in the areas of anesthesia...below the level of the SCI. It is variously described as tingling, aching, squeezing, throbbing, etc. The descriptions can be rather bizarre. Other problems can make central pain worse...infections, anxiety, depression, weather changes, etc. It is thought to be generated deep within the brain. It usually starts soon after the SCI and is found in about 33% of all SCI patients. There is no currently reliable treatment for this formidable pain syndrome. The treating physician will have to be persistent in trying to find a combination of medications that may work.

Secret Number 3: SCI treatment is directed mostly at a neuropathic mechanism. Lyrica, Cymbalta, and opiates are good choices for pain relief.

Spinal cord injury nerve pain is a challenge to treat. In the cases of SCI pain that I had in my practice of Pain Management, I found the discovery of the right combination of therapies took much persistence on both the part of my patients and myself. Yet and still, we eventually found an effective collection of treatments that would reduce the patient's pain.

VI. Psychological Pain Secrets

Munchausen Syndrome

Asher described the common features of his patients as:
- Repeatedly seeking admission into medical facilities under apparent physical or mental distress, offering plausible stories supporting the nature of their disorder.
- Once admitted, they may submit themselves to radical interventions.
- They leave against medical advice, often after exaggerated arguments with the medical staff.
- They later turn up in other facilities with the same or other phenomena
- Named syndrome after Baron von Munchausen.

Asher R. Munchausen's syndrome. Lancet 1951;1:339-341)

Why did Asher call it Munchausen syndrome?

There is a "pain" that affects a person so deeply that its origin cannot be found in simple diagnostic testing for a physical malady. All people who present to physicians with chronic pain are not necessarily experiencing a physical ailment. This section will be my attempt to introduce the group of psychiatric disorders that has been reclassified in the Diagnostic and Statistical Manual of Mental Disorders V (DSM-V) (published by the American Psychiatric Association) called Somatic Symptom Disorders.

As a retired Pain Management physician, I am reminded that, in addition to the challenge of correctly identifying the physical cause of a patient's chronic pain, there is a subset of patients that actually do not have a physical reason for their "pain". This does not necessarily mean that the patient is willfully dishonest.

The first well-described pattern of this type of patient was published by Dr. Richard Asher in 1951. He described a pattern of self-harm where a patient would fabricate their history, symptoms, and physical findings. The person had often traveled widely and was a dramatic story teller. Upon attempted verification of their dramatic stories, they were often found to have been lying or distorting the truth. Dr. Asher affectionately called the disorder "Munchausen's Syndrome" named after Baron von Munchhausen, a well-known storyteller from the 1700s. The Baron used to entertain guests at his home and tell colorful stories about his exploits. He became famous when a contemporary writer published a book about him using fantastic and impossible stories (fictionalized by the writer). Perhaps he intended to embarrass the Baron, but instead, made his name famous.

In Dr. Asher's rendition of "Munchausen's Syndrome," the affected person exaggerates or creates symptoms of illnesses in themselves to gain the attention and treatment of medical personnel. There is a peculiar and elusive type of psychopathology that underlies this type of behavior. The patient often succeeds in their efforts, therefore having unnecessary surgical procedures and often succumbing to the complications related to multiple surgeries. It is essential that medical doctors are aware of the risk that these patients pose to themselves and the medical licenses of those who treat them.

Secret Number 1: Somatic Symptom Disorders are not an uncommon form of mental illness.

The DSM-V calls these disorders, such as Munchausen's Syndrome, Somatic Symptom Disorders (SSD). These are a group of psychiatric disorders that have no organic or physical (somatic) cause for the bodily symptoms that the patient complains about. *I want to emphasize that simple dishonesty is not the only mechanism at work (though it could be in certain cases).* Unlike the classical dishonest person, many of these patients offer their symptoms at quite a physical cost to themselves without much practical gain. They often end up disabled and unproductive as a result of therapeutic misadventures. This category of disorders is not rare. It is estimated that they are the third leading cause of psychiatric illness (after Depression and Anxiety). Females seem to be at a much higher risk for this type of mental illness (almost a 10:1 female to male ratio). The overall incidence in the American population is estimated to be 12%.

The clues to an underlying SSD would be as follows:

- *Historical evidence of visiting multiple different medical practitioners.* Usually, they will not have one primary doctor that is coordinating their care.

- *There will be an anthology of medical diagnostic studies that will have been performed.* The studies will be without any abnormalities to explain their pain.

- *The history is usually dramatically explained by the SSD person.* There may be inferences that the other doctors simply "did not understand them" (despite having performed an extensive workup).

- *Any reference for a need to consider a psychiatric cause for their pain is usually met with disdain and dramatic refusal.*

- *There may be physical evidence of multiple surgical scars on physical examination.* Investigation of the

previous surgical findings will show no evidence of
abnormalities.

- *All objective findings for a physical cause for their
  pain will be negative.*

As you can see, convincing a person that there is no
physical explanation for their "pain" can be very
challenging. *Physicians rely on the accurate and honest
medical history of a patient to arrive at a proper
diagnosis. There is no diagnostic study that can replace
the accurate medical history on a patient.*

**Secret Number 2: There is no definitive test for Somatic
Symptom Disorder.**

There have been several recent reports in the
neuroscience literature that seem to indicate that brain
function in a person with an SSD is perturbed. It seems
that the neural connections between the front of the brain
(frontal cortex) and the amygdala (an almond sized portion
of the brain located deep in the temporal lobe) are poorly
developed. The amygdala is integral for processing
emotional information. The frontal cortex is essential for
processing information regarding impulse control and
decision making. Under development in these areas could
lead to inaccurate processing of emotional information,
impulsivity, and immaturity.

Why would a person feign chronic pain? What is to be gained? In some cases, there may be a motivation to obtain narcotic pain medicine. Most doctors would be loath to prescribe chronic pain medications without any objective findings on physical examination or diagnostic testing. The psychology of the SSD person is thought to be more complex than simple deception. This type of patient often has little in the way of a family support system. The SSD patient may be seeking emotional support and uses the physical presentation for the "secondary gain" from the emotional support of medical personnel. The actual psychological mechanism has not really been worked out. Much more scientific study is necessary for this very challenging group of psychiatric illnesses.

The mystery of psychological pain has yet to be understood. As you can imagine, well- controlled studies will be difficult to arrange given the nature of this type of psychiatric illness. What you cannot accurately study you will not be able to accurately treat. Somatic Symptom Disorders (which includes psychological pain) will need to be a priority for future study given the large number of people that are likely to develop this disorder.

Secret Number 3: Somatic Symptom Disorder may not be simple deception.

Chapter 7 – Secrets of the Complications of Chronic Pain

I. Secrets of the Sleep Disorder in Chronic Pain

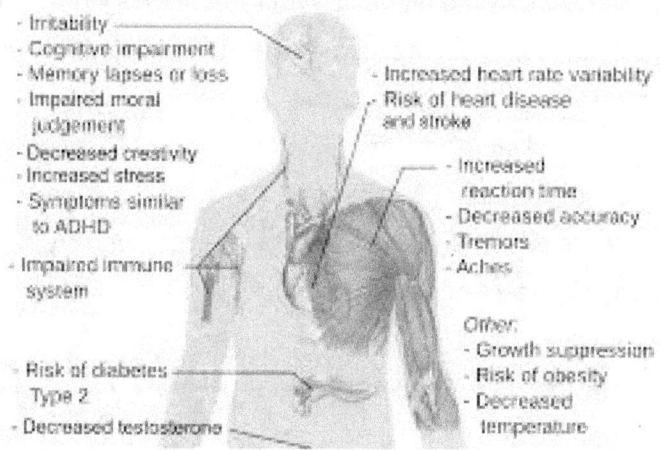

It has been said, "The next day begins the night before," and nowhere is this truer than in the case of sleep in human beings. The exact brain biochemistry for the restorative function of sleep has still to be discovered. And yet, go without sleep for much more than a week and most human beings will die.

The pattern of sleep for human beings falls into 3 types: 1) EARLY CHRONOTROPES ("early risers"), 2) MIDDLE CHRONOTROPES ("9 to 5ers"), and 3) LATE

CHRONOTROPES ("night owls"). The majority of people fall into the middle category. So there seems to be some innate, "God given," biochemical reason for sleep cycles in human beings. The electrical pattern in the most restful time of sleep (called REM sleep for "rapid eye movement") resembles the electrical pattern of being awake. Finally, a small structure in your brain called the Pineal Gland seems to help regulate your sleep pattern through a chemical called Melatonin. Multiple other areas of your brain are also involved in the process of sleep.

Secret Number 1: The brain never "sleeps" but changes its electrical activity during sleep.

The National Sleep Foundation puts the number of people with a sleep disorder in chronic pain at around 63% (this does not include people with acute pain). The combination of the pain, stress response, and depression seem to all play into the sleep disorder of chronic pain. Many pain practitioners will focus on inducing sleep when in fact the real need is to effectively treat a person's pain to re-establish their sleep pattern. Even then, many people with chronic pain will not establish a normal sleep pattern. This sleep disorder is thought to be the major reason for the increase in all-cause mortality in people with chronic pain. Yes, you heard me right, people with chronic pain live shorter lives and it is not just due to the underlying illnesses.

Secret Number 2: The increase in mortality of people in chronic pain is thought to be related to chronic sleep deprivation.

The first step in treating the sleep disorder with chronic pain is to have a complete history and physical by your primary care practitioner. Pending their review, a precise diagnosis must be made. You may need to see a Neurologist, who specializes in Sleep Disorders (or a Lung Specialist). Here are a few general suggestions to improve "sleep hygiene":

- Avoid all caffeine, nicotine, and other stimulants three hours before sleep.

- Avoid reading, watching television, or listening to the radio before sleep in your bedroom.

- Avoid over the counter sleep medications that use anti-histamines to induce sleep (the type of sleep that they produce is not restorative and not REM).

- Consider utilizing a sound generating device that may induce sleep (also known as "white noise").

- Remember to take your pain medications exactly as prescribed by your practitioner so that your pain is adequately controlled during sleep. You may need a supplemental dose of pain medicine at night as the blood level of your medicine may track low in a prolonged sleep interval.

Secret Number 3: Most difficulties with the sleep cycle in chronic pain come from inadequate treatment of the chronic pain.

If you suffer from a chronic pain sleep disorder, you will be able to establish a restful sleep cycle by following these simple guidelines. In most cases, your sleep cycle will not completely normalize even with treatment. Your goal should be to get sleep intervals of 4 hours or more with dreaming. This will reduce the negative physiologic effects of sleep deprivation.

II. Secrets of Sexual Dysfunction in Chronic Pain

CATEGORY	DISORDERS	PROBLEM
Psychogenic	Performance anxiety, Depression	Loss of libido, overinhibition, Impaired nitric oxide release
Neurogenic	Stroke, Spinal cord injury, Diabetic retinopathy	Lack of nerve impulse, or Interrupted transmission
Hormonal	Hypogonadism, Hyperprolactinoma	Inadequate nitric oxide release
Vasculogenic (arterial or venous	Atherosclerosis, hypertension	Impaired arterial or venous flow
Medication-induced	Antihypertensives, Antidepressants, Alcohol, cigarette use	Central suppression, Vascular insufficiency

A REAL CASE

Joseph (the name has been changed) shuffled into the examining room with a frown on his face. "Doc, I am in so much pain. Every minute of every day I have to deal with this pain in my abdomen. My surgeon thought it was my Gallbladder so he took it out...the pain continued. My Internist thought I had some type of psychiatric cause for my pain...so he referred me to a Psychiatrist, who medicated me so heavily that I was falling asleep driving my car. I still hurt anyways. And Doc...with all the pain...I haven't made love to my wife in 6 years. Could it get any worse for me?"

Secret Number 1: Nearly everyone with chronic pain has a sexual dysfunction of some type.

Joseph's complaint of sexual dysfunction was very common in my pain practice. Since chronic pain touches every aspect of a person's life, sexual dysfunction in a person with chronic pain should be no surprise. National statistics on sexual dysfunction in the United States ranges from 30 to 40 percent in people without chronic pain. Depending on the study you read, chronic pain patients have some sort of sexual dysfunction 60% of the time at the minimum.

I have never been a fan of sexual statistics. It's one of those topics that people have a hard time being totally honest about. In my clinical practice nearly every chronic pain patient had some type of problem with intimacy...if I was willing to listen and they were willing to tell me. **The physiologic response in human sexuality is complicated.** Human beings are complicated enough without having chronic pain, chronic pain medications, and the emotional response to chronic pain.

Secret Number 2: The sexual dysfunction in chronic pain is usually related to inadequate treatment of pain.

There are at least three basic mechanisms to disrupt human sexuality in people with chronic pain:

- *The most obvious is the very neurochemistry of pain.* Intractable pain raises cortisol, reduces dopamine, reduces serotonin, reduces norepinephrine, and reduces oxytocin. Normal levels of these neurotransmitters are essential to a "normal" sexual response.

- *The nature of the mechanism causing the pain.* Some chronic pain syndromes affect the very mechanics for human sexual response (i.e. chronic lumbar pain). Other chronic pain syndromes are directly related to intercourse and "torpedo" the intimacy (i.e. chronic pelvic pain).

- *The treatments for chronic pain can affect the human sexual response.* Opiate pain medications lower testosterone levels when taken long term. Certain surgeries can disrupt pelvic nerves literally disconnecting the sexual neural circuits.

Secret Number 3: The sexual dysfunction in chronic pain adds to the negative physiologic effect of the pain. Treatment of it not only restores hope but decreases the complication rate in chronic pain.

Thankfully, there are several important measures that can be taken to restore sexual function in a person with chronic pain:

- *First and foremost, treat the pain.* The likelihood that people with chronic pain will achieve a totally pain-free state is uncommon. However, predictable pain relief to a tolerable level (most people would report a "5" on a scale of 1 to 10 as tolerable) does wonders for a person's sexual response.

- *Understand the mechanism for the pain generation and devise a strategy to counteract its effect on the sexual response.*   For instance, if the person suffers from chronic hip pain, body positioning during sexual intercourse can reduce pain significantly. Discussions of this type are very private and require time with your pain practitioner.

- *Identify reversible sexual side effects of the treatments.* I used to run all the medications I was treating a person with through a side effect program that I kept on my IPhone (very handy in clinical practice).

In Joseph's case, his pain was treated with a "high tech" mechanism. I had a surgeon implant a long-lasting intravenous line in a large vein under his collar bone (the IV line is called a Hickman catheter). After his surgery, I started a continuous infusion of a synthetic narcotic called Nubain (this medication has a lower side effect profile but cannot be given by mouth) to be given by an external pump. He wore the pump as a "fanny pack" outside his body. In that way, I could easily adjust his pump rate by having him come into the office or by having an IV Nurse go to his home. He went home from the hospital with the apparatus. I had weaned him off of all his previous pain medications. His pain was down to a "5" for the first time in years.

When he returned to my office for his first post-hospitalization visit, he was smiling. He said," I made love to my wife for the first time in six years. You are the best, Doc." You couldn't wipe the smile off my face for a week. The Nubain had worked to relieve his pain with a minimum of side effects. He would need to be on the continuous pump for now...probably for years. **This** extreme measure was necessary because he could not tolerate the side effects of his pain medication given in any other manner. I had several people that required this type of pain therapy to maximize relief and minimize side effects.

If you suffer from sexual dysfunction, you will probably not have to resort to such extreme measures. A Pain Management physician should be able to identify the main reasons for your sexual dysfunction and correct them. There is hope for you...

III. Secrets of Chronic Pain and Fatigue

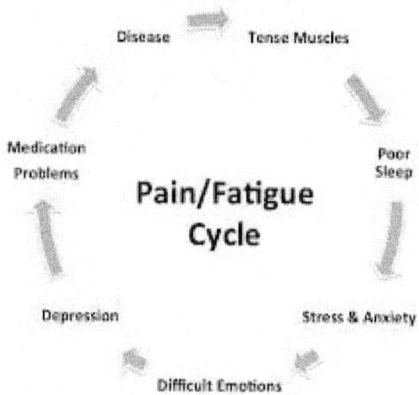

A REAL CASE

Mike's name was called three times in the waiting room by my office staff. No one waiting responded. My office manager saw a man asleep in the corner chair (on one of the soft sofas) and went over to him, "Excuse me sir, is your name Mike?" He opened his eyes, smiled, and followed her back into the examining room.

When I opened the exam room door, Mike started to talk immediately, "Doc, I am so tired that I don't want to get out of bed. I lost my job...my wife is frustrated with me...and we are about to lose our house in foreclosure. I have pain all the time and my Primary Care Physician (PCP) told me I just have to live with my pain. How am I to do that?" Mike is one of many people seen in clinical pain management practices dealing with chronic pain and fatigue. This complication of chronic pain is often over-looked by PCPs as they have so little time to interview patients these days.

Secret Number 1: Chronic fatigue associated with chronic pain is a sign that the physiology of the patient has worsened to the point of neurotransmitter exhaustion.

When a person suffers from the Chronic Pain Syndrome, they will often develop an overwhelming fatigue syndrome in addition to their pain. This can be a signal that they have begun to enter into the negative neurophysiologic changes that accompany the Chronic Pain Syndrome. Nearly all neurotransmitter production in the central and peripheral nervous system has a fixed maximal production capacity. Continual stimulation from chronic pain "outstrips" the production capacity of the neurons. When this happens secondary symptoms begin to occur…depression, insomnia, fatigue, etc. The usual approach many Doctors use is to treat each of these secondary symptoms as a separate illness. This only stresses the neurons further. It is akin to "whipping a horse" when it is exhausted…the horse may die before it gets to the finish line. A more physiologic approach would be to decrease the neurotransmitter "drain" and restore the supply.

Secret Number 2: The treatment of the chronic fatigue in chronic pain always requires that measures be taken to replace the low levels of neurotransmitters.

A pragmatic approach to the chronic pain patient with fatigue could be as follows:

A) Step 1: Reduce or eliminate the "drain" of neurotransmitters that is occurring. That may be accomplished in the following way:

1) Effectively treat a persons' pain. Most people who have deteriorated to the point that they are developing secondary symptoms from chronic pain can give you an estimate of what their pain medication needs would be. A Doctor can use their history of pain medicine effect to guide them as to what the starting dose of prescription pain medication should be. We do this with nearly all other medications, why not pain medicine?

2) *Establish what the sleep pattern of the person is.* Sleep deprivation in chronic pain patients is very common. When properly medicated for pain they will often have what is called "REM rebound" (they may sleep 2 or 3 times the length they usually would). This does not mean you are over-medicated. You are simply "catching up" on your sleep. You are, in effect, resupplying your neurotransmitters. This period of time is often misinterpreted by Doctors and family alike.

3) *A non-sedating anti-depressant in low doses may be started (preferably one that "recycles" both norepinephrine and serotonin).* An example of this would be a medication called Cymbalta.

4) *It may be necessary to start a low dose sleep medicine,* in the early phases of restoring the neurotransmitters, to initiate a more normal sleep pattern. The objective would be to use this short-term.

5) *It may also be necessary to use a low dose neuro-stimulant* during the waking hours to "push" the neurons so that you will be functional enough to return to work. The objective of this medication is also to be used short-term.

B) **Step 2: Gradually replenish the levels of neurotransmitters in the central and peripheral nervous system. This may be accomplished by:**

1) *Consider the nutraceutical regimen that was described in Chapter 5 in the section on Fibromyalgia.*

2) *Begin an exercise program that is water-based (low gravity effect) gradually increasing to land-based exercise.* The program would be best focused on building endurance gradually (this increases the number of energy generating organelles in your cells called mitochondria).

3) *Have a Consultation with an expert in Complementary and Alternative Medicine (CAM).* They will be able to fashion a nutraceutical and dietary regimen to enhance energy production.

4) *Have Phases 1 and 2 carefully supervised by your PCP.*

Secret Number 3: Exercise is the most physiologic way to enhance energy production. Graded exercise increases the number of mitochondria in most cells of your body. Mitochondria are the small organelles in cells that manufacture energy-rich molecules.

Mike went on to do well. He was able to follow many of the recommendations that were offered to him. Over a period of 12 months, he returned to work and was able to keep his home. He even took a second job for a period of time until his finances stabilized. If you are suffering as Mike did there is hope. You need to call your PCP and get started on your way to recovery. Show him or her this book to give them some ideas on how they may help you.

Remember that repletion of your neurotransmitters will take time (likely weeks). Your fatigue will decrease as the neurotransmitter levels return to normal. There is hope for you.

IV. Secrets of Chronic Pain and Addiction

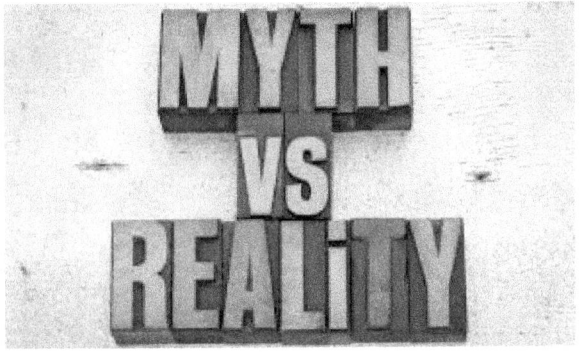

Chronic pain and addiction remain one of the most controversial areas in medicine today. There is still a misunderstood belief that the use of prescription pain medication for chronic pain (particularly opioid pain medications) "makes" a person an addict.

This is still stubbornly believed by patients and Doctors alike. However, the incidence of opiate addiction in the United States is 3% – 16 %...a statistic that has not changed since the Civil War. Also, what is to be done about people who have been addicts and have chronic pain? Are they disqualified from prescription pain medicine? Are people who are alcoholics, mentally unstable, or use marijuana also disqualified? In today's predatory prosecution of pain management physicians, these issues will not be objectively addressed. Also, the fear of legal reprisal de-motivates Doctors who are already ambivalent about chronic pain medications.

Secret Number 1: The only way to reliably tell whether a person is having addictive complications is to follow them while taking their medications.

Unfortunately, the medical history of a person who has never been an addict is unreliable as an indicator of how a person will do on chronic pain medication. No psychological, neurological, or sociological history can predict whether a person with chronic pain will become addicted to chronic pain medications. Openness and honesty in the Doctor – Patient relationship is essential **as the Doctor is not a prophet.** Remember, not treating chronic pain has inherent risks too (early death from suicide, heart attack, stroke, etc.).

The ethnic background, appearance, number of tattoos, muscularity, beard configuration, etc. have all been shown to not correlate with whether a person becomes addicted to their prescription pain medications or not. There has never been a physical finding that predicts whether a person on chronic pain medication will become addicted. The many biases in this area have never been proven by scientific studies.

Secret Number 2: ***There are no "risk-free" treatment options in chronic pain management.***

So what is the Doctor who wants to show compassion and treat his patient to do? I am going to suggest the following sensible guidelines:

- *First prove that the person has been correctly diagnosed with a disorder that would cause chronic pain.* This will usually have required a "workup" that included a thorough History and Physical, Diagnostic studies, and often a subspecialist's consultation. Unfortunately, all the studies that are presently used to determine the cause of pain do not actually measure whether a patient is experiencing pain and how much. Pain is physiologic and the studies used to justify the use of opiate pain medicines are structural measures. It would be like looking at the picture of an oven and deciding how hot it is. You have to be able to measure the heat to know the temperature. There is no such measure available for pain.

- An assessment of the psychological state of the hurting patient. There are also no reliable methods to do this easily. The evidence of active addictive behavior would be the only caution to adding another habituating medicine.

- A narcotic contract is presented to the person that outlines expectations for the relationship between the treating Doctor and the patient taking the pain medication. It will usually require regular urine drug screening, regular visits, and a single physician to prescribe the pain medications.

- *The pain level of the patient should be documented at each visit (the "1 to 10" pain scale is the standard).* When a patient is deceptive it will be difficult for them to remember all the previous pain ratings they have given their pain management provider.

- *The patient should be given an opportunity for a "probationary period" to see how they handle the medications.* Having an available quantity of pain medicine for a patient in pain is a set-up for non-compliance. Early "overuse" of the medicine would be expected with most patients.

- *A reassessment should be done shortly after the probationary period begins.*

- *Openness and honesty on the part of the patient are essential for correct assessment of their response to medications. Many pain patients will be reticent to be too open for fear of losing the medicine which is giving them relief.*

*Secret Number 3: It is not more righteous to leave a
patient in pain to avoid addiction.*

There must be more grace in how we approach the "brain
disorder" called addiction. Is it not curious that, despite
the "war on drugs", the incidence of drug addiction has
not changed since 1865? During the Vietnam War, it is
estimated that 20% of the returning soldiers were actively
using Heroin while they were on their military tour.
However, 98% of those same soldiers stopped using
Heroin when they returned to their homes in the U.S.
They did not have to enter a drug rehabilitation program
to do this. The effect of returning to stable families and
communities was enough to counter persistent, addictive
behavior. If it was simply the use of a habituating
substance that "creates an addict" we should have seen
the persistent use of Heroin when the soldiers returned to
the U.S. from Vietnam.

In medicine the Doctors creed had always been..." Cure
occasionally...Treat most...and comfort always". Is it
possible we could return to this as our "prime
directive"? **If you are on chronic pain medications, you are
not automatically an addict. You are a person with chronic
pain and one of the most predictable ways to relieve your
pain is with the prescription medications you are taking.
Addiction is synonymous to obsession. Obsession is not a
pharmacologic phenomenon.**

VII. Secrets of the Overwhelming Effect of Pain on the Person

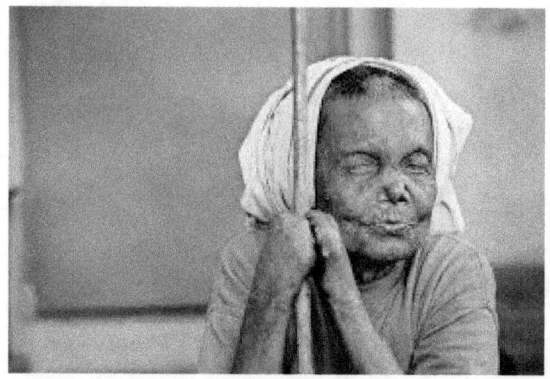

"And the leper in whom the plague is, his clothes shall be rent, and his head bare, and he shall put a covering upon his upper lip, and shall cry, Unclean, unclean. All the days wherein the plague shall be in him he shall be defiled; he is unclean: he shall dwell alone, without the camp shall his habitation be." Leviticus 13: 45-46 The Holy Bible, KJV

The purpose of this chapter will be to help you enhance your understanding of the impact that chronic pain has, on the whole person. I believe that the metaphor using leprosy as a symbolic comparison to the "leper of today" ...the chronic pain patient...fits appropriately. Leprosy is a disease that was feared among the ancients. It was reported as early as 600 BC in India, China, and Egypt. It is an infectious disease that deforms the face, fingers, toes, ears, nose and elsewhere (see the above picture). It also degenerates the nerves causing anesthesia of the areas it infects. The exact mode of transmission is still unknown. It doesn't kill directly but lingers for years causing disfigurement of its victims.

Secret Number 1: Chronic pain patients often feel like they are treated like modern day lepers.

Chronic pain, like Leprosy, affects every aspect of a person's life. The medical condition itself is only one aspect of the pervasive effect the disease has upon a person. Chronic pain is defined as daily pain that lasts for three or more months. Whereas acute pain is an early warning system that alerts one to a physical problem, chronic pain has no such beneficial alert. The very physiology of acute pain uses a different segment of your nervous system from what chronic pain uses.

Chronic pain affects areas of the body remote from the location where the pain is being generated. For instance, a person with chronic back pain can be expected to have difficulty sleeping, difficulty with sexual intimacy, difficulty concentrating, difficulty with depression... all effects remote to the source of the pain.

Chronic pain offers no apparent benefit to a human being. The incidence of many causes of death is increased in the presence of chronic pain. People with heart disease die sooner with chronic pain, even given the same severity of heart disease than a person without chronic pain. The incidence of cancer, strokes, and psychiatric illness are all higher in people with chronic pain. Chronic pain is an amplifier of the negative.

RELATIONSHIPS ARE AFFECTED...

In my practice, I was able to observe the cumulative effects of chronic pain on relationships. Let's face it...chronic pain affects how we relate to each other. A stable long term relationship can be seriously affected when one member has chronic pain. The sexual intimacy of that relationship is not only affected but its emotional intimacy is too. The distraction of the chronic pain causes apathy towards intimacy. The interest in putting the effort forth for emotional intimacy wanes when one's energy is depleted by constant pain.

It doesn't take long for a couple to develop separate, parallel lifestyles in the presence of chronic pain. Life must go on whether both parties can participate equally or not. The pain- free partner often seeks their emotional needs to be filled elsewhere...further deepening the emotional crevasse that exists.

FINANCIAL SECURITY IS AFFECTED...

Not only does chronic pain reduce the ability of a person to be gainfully employed but it also increases the medical expenditures by a person. Multiple doctor visits, procedures, hospitalizations, medications, special medical equipment, special therapies, and rehabilitation exhaust medical insurance coverage.

Eventually, if not effectively treated, many chronic pain patients will require financial assistance and governmental insurance coverage. Their ability to generate enough income to cover their health expenses is limited. Unless very financially secure before the onset of their chronic pain syndrome, they often become financially destitute. The need for the extended family to supplement the income of the chronic pain patient becomes necessary...a tricky development to navigate in a culture where families are fragmenting daily.

EMOTIONAL HEALTH IS AFFECTED...

The person with chronic pain has their emotional health shredded. In addition to their personal self-esteem being affected, they see the "drain" they have become upon their family. Men are particularly prone to this effect and have a much higher incidence of violent suicidal attempts when they suffer from chronic pain.

Secret Number 2: The incidence of suicide in chronic pain patients is under-reported.

Death certificate analysis for cause of death in chronic pain patients is notoriously inaccurate as doctors fill out death certificates with the consideration of legal reprisal and life insurance benefits. It is much more "tidy" to report the death of a chronic pain patient as an "accidental overdose" than to report it as "ineffective treatment of pain". The guilt that follows for the living is more easily negotiated with this type of inaccurate reportage. Also, insurance companies ask fewer questions...as do legal authorities.

For those who "soldier on" in their chronic pain...depression is the rule. Doctors often treat the depression as the primary problem. What is really necessary is to treat the person's pain effectively. Chronic pain causes personality changes that reduce the likelihood that important relationships will endure. The person with chronic pain is distracted, inattentive, withdrawn, depressed, unmotivated, and generally uninterested in the activities necessary to maintain emotional intimacy with others.

SOCIAL INTERACTION IS AFFECTED...

The social structure of a patient in chronic pain eventually deteriorates. Unable to engage in family gatherings, religious activities, social events, etc. the pain patient becomes a social non-entity. Their name is eventually forgotten and they are not included in the usual activities...an "out of sight...out of mind" phenomena.

Not to mention that the chronic pain sufferer may not have the stamina to be socially engaged. The many questions about their condition, the medications they are taking, and the proverbial "have you tried..." (An assertion that is often interpreted by a person in chronic pain as a question of the legitimacy of their pain).

It may also be that the presence of a person in chronic pain at a social event is a reminder of one's own enlightened self-interest. A psychological realization that causes too much self-reflection for the pain-free population. The lack of real involvement in a family member's chronic pain is a reminder of our own shallowness. Who wants to be reminded of that?

RELIGIOUS FAITH IS TESTED...

If you had a theology of a loving God before you developed a chronic pain syndrome...upon developing chronic pain, it will be tested. The proverbial "well God has a plan for your pain..." is not usually very comforting to a person in chronic pain. There can be no doubt that more acts of righteousness towards one another are done in the face of suffering. We just don't seem to have a natural love one for another when things are going well for us. Perhaps humans need to see others suffer to show sacrificial love for each other. It is curious that the founders of most relief organizations have been personally affected by suffering before having the vision to set up their organization.

THE BLEAKNESS OF SUFFERING ALONE...

As my final observation, the one I believe to be "the mother of all impacts in chronic pain," is the most poignant to me. It is the bleakness of suffering alone. In this final insight I think the treatment of lepers is particularly relevant. Far surpassing the disfigurement, the broken relationships, the shredded self-image of the leper, and the poverty...they are forced to go it alone. There was no gentle touch, support group, or fellowship for the leper. He was outside the camp...infrequently visited no doubt.

Secret Number 3: Most chronic pain patients experience significant isolation.

So it goes with the chronic pain person. Frequently stigmatized by the way they look, smell, medications they take, how their home may look...chronic pain patients often suffer alone. *Doctors avoid them, nurses deride them, pharmacies spurn them, law enforcement ridicules them...the chronic pain person is a modern day leper.* They suffer without the comfort of others and they often live in isolation. Those who show compassion to the person in chronic pain may suffer a similar social ostracism (a form of guilt by association).

It doesn't have to be this way for those in chronic pain. Those of us fortunate enough to be pain-free can begin to reach out today. We each know someone who would appreciate a phone call, a text message, an email, a letter...or perhaps even a visit. One act of kindness goes a long way with a person who is suffering alone. The mere knowledge that others are concerned about you can fuel an attitude change in a person who is suffering. Don't be afraid to reach out to the leper...

"Then shall the King say unto them on his right hand, Come, ye blessed of my Father, inherit the kingdom prepared for you from the foundation of the world: For I was hungered, and ye gave me meat: I was thirsty, and ye gave me drink: I was a stranger, and ye took me in: Naked, and ye clothed me: I was sick, and ye visited me: I was in prison, and ye came unto me."

Matthew 25:34-36, <u>The Holy Bible</u>, KJV

Chapter 8 – Secrets of the Common Treatments for Chronic Pain

I. Opiate Medication Secrets

There are few more controversial topics in the field of medicine than the legitimate use of prescription pain medications for chronic non-malignant pain. Everyone has an opinion...and they are usually very earnest in their point of view. Why does the "crevasse" that separates the groups exist? It's complicated...

Secret Number 1: The specific differences in treating acute pain versus chronic pain have not been taught in most medical school curricula.

Most residencies do not offer clinical training in chronic pain management. It seems inconceivable that chronic pain, a syndrome that every Doctor will encounter, would not be taught. But it isn't... To add insult to injury, the "war on drugs" by the U.S. Federal Government has resulted in the targeting of pain management physicians (much "softer" targets than violent drug cartels) who treat pain with large doses of prescription pain medications. This has resulted in many physicians under treating their patient's pain for fear of legal reprisal. The issue seems to have gone "sideways".

There are many myths in the field of chronic pain management so I have selected four that I think would be of greatest interest to people:

Myth Number 1: "I must be addicted if I have withdrawal symptoms when I stop my prescription pain medications."

The human body is a complex integrated wonder. Axiomatic to its function is the idea of "negative feedback". What that simply means is that what is low will be made to come up and vice versa. Did you know you can "withdraw" from certain high blood pressure medications? Do an internet search on Catapres (a hypertension medication) and you may be surprised that there is a withdrawal syndrome if it is abruptly discontinued. Your body will "adapt" to any medicine that is presented to it regularly.

Secret Number 2: The normal response to taking a pain medication every day is to require more over time and become dependent on it. This is not addiction.

Myth Number 2: "If I take my prescription pain medication long enough I will become addicted."

There is confusion in the use of the word "addiction" among health care practitioners and many others. Addiction is a chronic syndrome that is a compulsion to take a substance despite severe dysfunction with its continued use. Dependency is a physiologic phenomenon that has no compulsive qualities. People who take prescription pain medications all become dependent (with a minority becoming compulsive or addicted). For that matter, if you are on a traditionally non-addicting medication on a chronic basis there is a strong likelihood you will become dependent on it (but not addicted).

Myth Number 3: "It is better to live with my pain than to risk addiction."

When it comes to chronic pain management, there is no "risk-free" option. People who have untreated chronic pain are at much higher risk of death from suicide, cardiac disease, stroke, cancer, and a variety of other illnesses.

Chronic pain wounds a person and sets them up for other diseases. Treating chronic pain lowers the risk of dying from these other diseases, not to mention that it shows compassion on the part of the Doctor.

Myth Number 4: "My doctor will just naturally know if I become addicted to my prescription pain medication."

In order for your Doctor to help you from developing any complication from a prescribed medicine, you will need to be completely honest about how you are doing. The honesty in the "Doctor-Patient Relationship" is the best way to identify problems that can develop. Could you imagine a Doctor trying to make an accurate diagnosis and the patient lied about their symptoms? The integrity of the relationship is essential to its effectiveness. Doctors are not prophets...

Under the best circumstances, taking prescription pain medication is tricky. Most people with chronic pain who are on prescribed medications will do well. Maintain an open and honest dialogue with the Doctor, have regular follow-up visits, and take the medication exactly as prescribed. You will obtain relief from your pain.

Secret Number 3: Doctors are not prophets and need help in determining whether a patient has become addicted to their pain medicine.

II. Motrin (Ibuprofen) Secrets

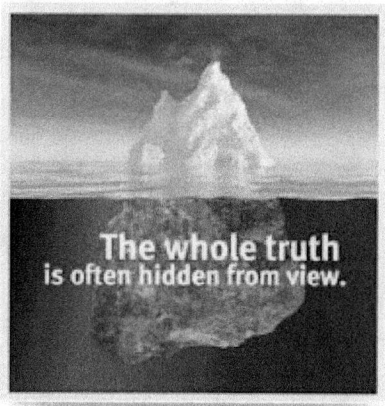

Motrin is an effective anti-pain and anti-fever medicine. Along with the beneficial effects of this medicine come many natural risks. NON-STEROIDAL ANTI-INFLAMMATORY drugs (or NSAIDs for short) is the general category of medication that Motrin falls into. Most of the statistics for NSAIDs have been collected using prescription data. This is because it is much easier to retrieve prescription data for experimental study due to the careful documentation that Doctors and Pharmacists must keep when prescribing and dispensing these medicines.

HISTORY OF MOTRIN

Motrin was originally developed in 1961 by the Boots Company in the United Kingdom. The intention was to develop another NSAID that was safer than large doses of aspirin. It was introduced into the U.K in 1966 and the U.S. in 1974. It was originally available by prescription only. However, by 1984 it was available over-the-counter (OTC) in both countries. The actual usage patterns of Motrin are estimates based on the prescription dispensing statistics

I think it is reasonable to say that the reported incidence of side effects for these medications are woefully under-recognized due to the OTC status of the medicine. There is, as yet, no systematic way to track the case by case use of OTC medications. Unbeknownst to the world there is a "silent epidemic" of toxic side effects that is being caused by the abundant use of NSAIDs OTC and by prescription. Furthermore, the under-reporting of the side effects of NSAIDs is occurring while mostly taking the medicines as recommended. The toxic side effects of NSAIDs are generally not due to overdoses.

This issue gets even more complicated. The estimate of the side effects of any medicine need to be measurable and directly related to the use of the medicine in question. However, the problem with NSAIDs is they can exert their toxic influence by the worsening of a person's primary disease. What do I mean by this? It has become very apparent that the higher the dose of an NSAID the greater the negative effect it has on heart disease. If a person taking NSAIDs dies suddenly from a heart condition, what does their death certificate likely say? In most cases, the death will be attributed to the underlying heart disease and not the NSAID. The contribution of the NSAID to the person's death is easily overlooked because the toxic effect is to worsen the underlying heart disease. Also, remember that we are talking about prescription drug data. What about someone taking an OTC NSAID who dies from a heart attack? Would anyone even recognize the association? Probably not...so I think you can see my caution in using this category of medicines. I believe that they represent the greater threat to the public's health than other more commonly publicized medications.

Secret Number 1: Motrin can have a toxic effect on people with pre-existing heart disease, even when used in the proper way and properly dosed.

THE NSAID MECHANISM

The human body has a series of chemical messengers that it utilizes to transfer information and initiate physiologic functions. Hormones are chemical messengers that can travel in the bloodstream as well as remain in one local area. Prostaglandins are local hormones (for the most part). Prostaglandins occupy local sites in body tissue and activate certain chemical messaging. Certain prostaglandins (PGs) cause your temperature to go up and others cause it to go down. Furthermore, certain PGs increase blood flow by opening or relaxing blood

191 | P a g e

vessels...others do the reverse. Your local hormones are in a balance (like most functions in a healthy human body). In the case of Motrin, the PGs that increase body temperature and pain are reduced by blocking enzymatic conversion. This makes Motrin a very effective pain medicine and fever reducer. When fever and pain are primarily mediated by PGs, Motrin can actually be more effective than Tylenol.

MOTRIN INDICATIONS

The following is a partial listing of the conditions Motrin may be good for (notice it is the exact same list as for Tylenol):

- Tension Headache

- Migraine Headache

- Toothache pain

- Temporomandibular Joint Syndrome

- Earache pain

- Neck Pain

- Back Pain

- Carpel Tunnel Syndrome

- Degenerative Joint Disease

- Rheumatoid Arthritis pain

- Knee pain

- Hip pain

- Plantar Fasciitis pain

- Ankle Sprain and Strain pain

- Menstrual pain

- Kidney Stone pain

- Costochondritis pain

- Pain Associated with Simple Bruises

- Fever

MOTRIN DOSING

The usual effective adult dose for Motrin varies from 200 milligrams very four to six hours as needed to 800 milligrams every six hours (the absolute maximum allowable dose). Doses above 800 milligrams every six hours have not been shown to be more effective in treatment and have a radical increase in toxic side effects (this is called a "ceiling effect"). Taking your Motrin with food may reduce some of the gastro-intestinal side effects but not the cardiovascular side effects. Dosing Motrin for children requires an adjustment according to weight and age. I refer you to the many published tables for doing this. This present book is primarily directed at treating chronic pain in adults.

MOTRIN SIDE EFFECTS

Motrin is a safely used medication when properly appreciated for its toxic side effects. There is an old saying, "any drug of any positive effect must have side effects." There is no way to take Motrin without risk (as is true with all medicines and surgeries). I would like you to appreciate a few things about this excellent medication:

1) NSAIDs increase the risk of death:

The number of people dying from NSAID-related complications (remember this number is conservative) actually exceeds the number of soldiers that died in the peak year of the Vietnam War. It also exceeds the number of people who die being murdered by firearms each year.

2) NSAIDs increase the likelihood that a person will be hospitalized.

3) The second most commonly prescribed NSAID is Motrin (after Celebrex). When combined with the OTC use it exceeds all other NSAIDs used by people.

Secret Number 2: NSAIDs are responsible for nearly 17,000 deaths each year due to gastro-intestinal

hemorrhage. This number is a conservative estimate since it depends on prescription statistics and does not include OTC use. This statistic does not include deaths by stroke and heart attacks that may be induced by NSAIDS.

4) Motrin has an extensive side effect profile.

The following side effects have been associated with the use of Motrin (and this is an incomplete listing):

- Stroke
- ringing in your ears
- rash
- mild itching
- nervousness
- dizziness
- constipation
- diarrhea
- bloating/gas
- nausea/vomiting
- heartburn
- upset stomach
- Heart Attack

- Gastro-intestinal Hemorrhage

- Stroke

5) Motrin has a dangerous pregnancy rating when taken after 30 weeks of pregnancy (Category D).

Before 30 weeks the pregnancy rating is Category C. Usually only Categories A to C are prescribed during pregnancy.

Secret Number 3: The Category D pregnancy rating makes Motrin unsuitable for use in pregnancy.

6) Motrin has 405 Drug interactions of which 96 are serious.

 If you are taking any other medicine or supplement, it is imperative that you have your pharmacist perform a drug interaction check before you take Motrin.

IN CONCLUSION...

I hope after reading this section you can see that even OTC Motrin is a serious medicine. You can take it safely if you do so under the guidance of your primary care practitioner. OTC medicine must always be considered when you are taking prescription medications due to the interactive effect between them. Any medicine of a clinical effect always has side effects.

III. Tylenol Secrets

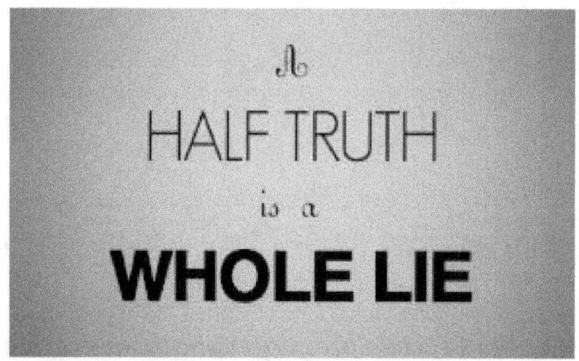

So if a medicine is over-the-counter (OTC) it must be safe, right? Well...what about those news reports of potential liver toxicity, kidney toxicity, skin toxicity, toxicity to the fetus, overdose emergency room visits, and hospitalizations all related to Tylenol? You might wonder how it ever became legal. In actuality, Tylenol is very safe when taken as directed. Be careful making decisions about therapies (or anything else for that matter) based on the sensationalized reports by our news media. I had used Tylenol extensively in my Pain Medicine practice and never had any serious side effects in any patients that took it as directed.

TYLENOL HISTORY

The American generic name for Tylenol is acetaminophen. Canada, Japan and a few other countries with close ties to the U.S. also use the same generic name. However, the predominately used international name is paracetamol. The chemical name "American style" is N-**acet**yl-p-**aminophen**ol (also called APAP). The name acetaminophen is a shortened hybrid of the chemical name. Tylenol is the number one used OTC pain medicine in the U.S.

The first development of this substance was in 1852 by Charles Gerhardt, a French chemist. It was called acetanilide. In 1899, Karl Morner (a German scientist) discovered that acetanilide was metabolized in the liver to the active compound acetaminophen. The actual production of the direct compound came years later. However, widespread use did not occur until McNeil Laboratories (headquartered in Philadelphia, Pennsylvania at the time) marketed APAP with Butabarbital as a prescription pain relieving medicine in 1953. Shortly after that, Children's Tylenol was released on the market by the same company (in 1955). It was offered as a safer alternative to aspirin for children. In 2005 over 28 billion doses of Tylenol (or Tylenol combined with another medicine) were used by Americans.

TYLENOL MECHANISM

One would think that for the long period of time Tylenol has been around that we would have a detailed understanding of how it works...we don't. We do know that it works on a category of chemical messengers called prostaglandins. These local hormones modulate the transmission of pain signaling and the production of a fever response in illness or injury. By blocking the prostaglandins, pain and fever can be blocked. This puts Tylenol in a category of medicines called NSAIDs (or non-steroidal anti-inflammatory medicines).

Secret Number 1: Tylenol is not associated with the same incidence of gastro-intestinal hemorrhage, stroke, or heart attack as with other NSAIDs.

Although it is in the same class as aspirin and ibuprofen (Motrin), Tylenol does not affect the prostaglandin system in the same way. A very good difference is that the formation of stomach ulcers is not seen with Tylenol. Furthermore, the clotting problems seen with aspirin and ibuprofen do not occur with Tylenol. All good news for Tylenol (and McNeil Laboratories).

TYLENOL INDICATIONS

Tylenol is a very good medicine for pain and fever relief. The following in a partial listing of the conditions Tylenol may be good for (notice it is the exact same list as Motrin):

- Tension Headache

- Migraine Headache

- Toothache pain

- Temporomandibular Joint Syndrome

- Earache pain

- Neck Pain

- Back Pain

- Carpel Tunnel Syndrome

- Degenerative Joint Disease

- Rheumatoid Arthritis pain

- Knee pain

- Hip pain

- Plantar Fasciitis pain

- Ankle Sprain and Strain pain

- Menstrual pain

- Kidney Stone pain

- Costochondritis pain

- Pain Associated with Simple Bruises

- Fever

TYLENOL DOSING

Tylenol is taken every four to six hours as an adult. It comes in 325 mg and 500 mg strengths. The total daily adult dose of Tylenol should not exceed 4000 mg. In people over 65 years of age or with liver malfunction the top dose of 2500 mg per day or less is recommended. The dosing for children requires adjustment according to age and weight.

Normal dosing of Tylenol can have side effects. A good "rule of thumb" to follow with side effects is, "any negative change in condition after starting Tylenol requires immediate stopping of the medicine and evaluation by a licensed primary care practitioner or physician."

Secret Number 2: Tylenol has a "ceiling effect" of 4000 mg per day in the adult population.

TYLENOL SIDE-EFFECTS

People with pre-existing liver or kidney disease should only take Tylenol under the direct supervision of a licensed primary care practitioner or physician. That includes a history of alcoholism, drug abuse, and Hepatitis (any type). You must also be very aware of the medications you are taking and any interaction that may occur with Tylenol. The direction of your primary care practitioner or physician is essential to properly evaluate drug interactions. Tylenol has over 160 different medications that it may interact with. Special conditions such as pregnancy and nursing are also times to be very careful taking it. There have been reports of a higher incidence of Asthma in children of mothers having taken Tylenol during their pregnancy.

IN CONCLUSION

The use of Tylenol can be very safe and effective for chronic pain. There have been comparisons made of its pain relieving properties to be equivalent to morphine (in terms of pain relief – 1300mg of Tylenol is equivalent to 4 mg of Morphine in pain relief). I always recommend that initial Tylenol use (especially OTC) be supervised by a licensed medical practitioner. It is a powerful medicine despite it being available over the counter.

Secret Number 3: Tylenol 1300 mg is equivalent to 4 mg of Morphine in pain relieving effect.

IV. Therapeutic Exercise Secrets

I know, it seems crazy, you are having chronic low back pain and you are being told that you need to exercise. You would probably think it makes more sense to get rid of your pain first and then you will exercise. In point of fact, exercise for chronic low back pain is like taking medicine.

THE MECHANISM OF PAIN RELIEF WITH EXERCISE

The following mechanisms are evoked with exercise to decrease pain:

1) Chronic low back pain is often caused by inflammation. There are substances called CYTOKINES that modulate inflammation. When we exercise, we decrease the levels of these substances. It is like taking aspirin without having to worry about getting an ulcer.

2) Naturally occurring substances in your brain called ENDORPHINES work just like morphine. When you exercise your brain releases these substances and relieves your pain.

3) Exercise increases blood flow and oxygen to muscles, ligaments, tendons, and nerves in your lower back. This facilitates healing and growth of new tissue which reduces pain.

Secret Number 1: There are at least 3 mechanisms that reduce pain with exercise.

WHAT EXERCISES ARE THE MOST EFFECTIVE?

The following seven exercises for chronic low back pain have been found to be very effective in relieving pain:

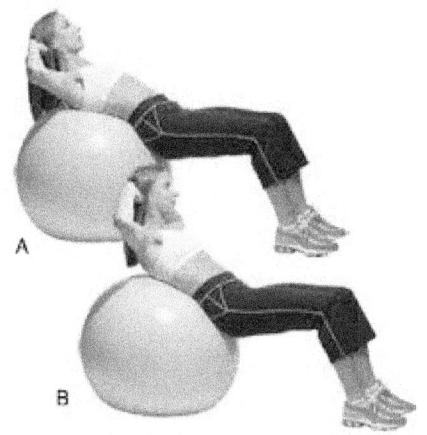

A

B

1) **Partial Crunches:** These are done instead of sit-ups (which are really bad for a person with back pain...so much for my grade school gym teacher). Lying on your back on an exercise ball (this can be done on a mat without the ball), tighten your abdominal muscles and raise your shoulders (to about 45 degrees). Hold in that position about one second then lower back down. Repeat this eight to 12 times. Strengthening your abdominal muscles increases your CORE strength which supports your back. Partial Crunches are great for your core (and back).

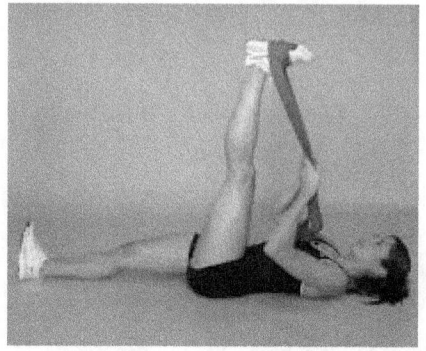

2) **Hamstring Stretches:** these are also done while lying on your back. Take a towel...loop it around one foot...and pull back on the towel while straightening that leg. Hold in that position for 15 to 30 seconds. Do that two to four times on each leg alternating. This exercise stretches an important nerve running down the back of your leg called the sciatic nerve (often pinched in low back pain).

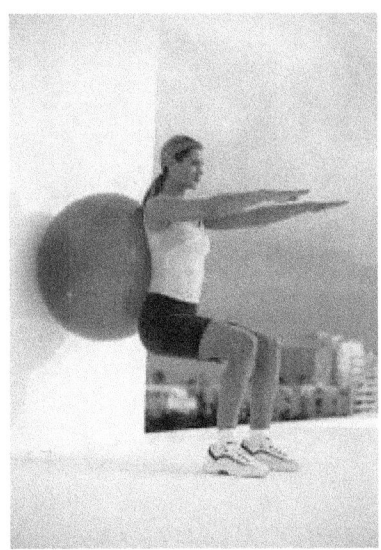

3) **Wall Sits:** Stand with an exercise ball against a wall (you can do this without the ball just pressing your back against the wall). Then, slowly lower yourself sliding down the wall until your knees are bent 65 to 90 degrees. Hold for a 10 count then slide back up. Repeat this movement eight to 12 times. This exercise braces your back while exercising it.

Secret Number 2: Exercises for back pain do not increase the axial load on the back (compressing the spine).

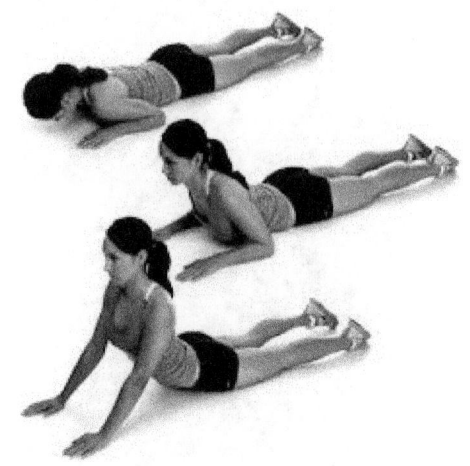

4) **Press-up Back Extensions:** While lying on a mat on
your belly...push up with your arms (your forearms will be
resting on the mat). This will cause your lower back to arch
and stretch. Hold for a count of five then lower back
down. Repeat the maneuver eight to 12 times. Arching
your lower back stretches it without putting a great deal of
strain on it.

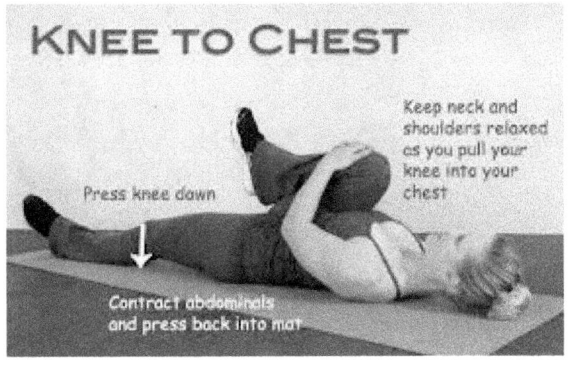

5) **Knee to Chest:** Again while lying on your back...pull one leg up to your chest (bending the knee). Keep your lower back pressed to the mat. Hold that position for a 15 count then lower that leg and repeat the motion with your other leg. Do this two to four times with each leg.

Secret Number 3: Exercises for back pain stretch the back structure acting like a form of muscular traction.

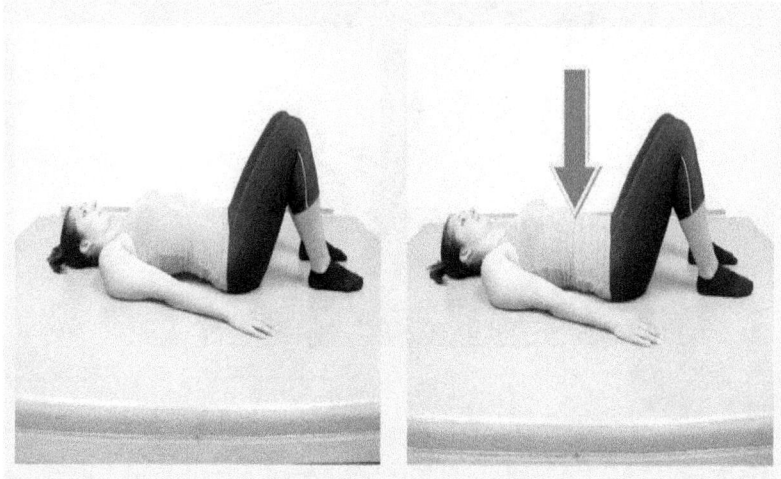

6) **Pelvic Tilts:** Lying on the mat...feet flat on the mat and legs bent at the knees...push your lower back flat against the mat. Hold that position for 10 seconds...repeat eight to 12 times.

7) **Aquacise:** I have added this to "best exercises" for a couple reasons. I know that it may not be convenient because you are going to have to find a pool that has classes. But, the effort will be worth it. The buoyancy of the water has an anti-gravity effect. This takes a lot of strain off your lower back. Furthermore, the water adds some resistance to any exercise you might do. You will also have the benefit of the cooling effect of being in the water (it is almost impossible to overheat during aquacise).

IN CONCLUSION

If you are suffering from chronic low back **pain,** you need
to take exercise out of the "optional category" and place it
in the "mandatory category." Exercise is "medicine" for a
person in chronic pain. **Begin your "medicine" today and
start exercising.** Begin with the exercises we have
suggested after consulting with your Doctor. What do you
have to lose other than some pain? Remember, any
exercise program you may initiate should be done under
the guidance of a licensed medical practitioner. There is
hope for your pain with an exercise program tailored to
your specific needs.

**V. Osteopathic Manipulative Therapy (Chiropractic
Therapy) Secrets**

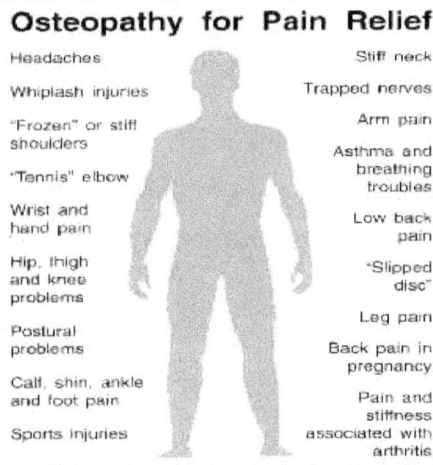

Osteopathy for Pain Relief

Headaches

Whiplash injuries

"Frozen" or stiff
shoulders

"Tennis" elbow

Wrist and
hand pain

Hip, thigh
and knee
problems

Postural
problems

Calf, shin, ankle
and foot pain

Sports injuries

Stiff neck

Trapped nerves

Arm pain

Asthma and
breathing
troubles

Low back
pain

"Slipped
disc"

Leg pain

Back pain in
pregnancy

Pain and
stiffness
associated with
arthritis

When the discussions about Osteopathic Manipulative Therapy or Chiropractic treatment for spinal pain are entertained there seems to always be a strong opinion. It is almost like having a discussion about religion or politics. Some people "swear" by this type of treatment and others swear at it. Osteopathic Manipulative Therapy and Chiropractic Manipulative Therapy have become synonymous with Spinal Manipulative Therapy (SMT).

THE HISTORY OF SPINAL MANIPULATIVE THERAPY

Chiropractors are not the only medical professionals that perform SMT. Osteopathic physicians (medical initials D.O.), M.D.s, and Physical Therapists may all become trained in SMT. The history of SMT dates back to 1872 when an M.D. physician by the name of Dr. Andrew Taylor Still set up the first school of Osteopathic Medicine in Kirksville, Missouri. He left the traditional field of medicine after his wife and 3 children died from spinal meningitis. His medical school changed the professional designation for its graduates from M.D. to D.O. (Doctor of Osteopathy). His graduates were taught all the usual information taught in medical school along with his new visionary approach to the inter-relationship of the spine and health of the body.

Secret Number 1: SMT has been practiced for over 140 years.

Dr. Still originated many of the SMT techniques still in use today. He was a pioneer in understanding spinal anatomy and physiology. One of Dr. Still's students was the founder of Chiropractic. In 1895, Daniel David Palmer set up the first school of Chiropractic Medicine. He had been a student with Dr. Still for only 6 weeks and left the program at Kirksville. The actual history about this is scant. Dr. Still is rarely mentioned in the history of Chiropractic Medicine. It is because of this common origin that Osteopathic Medicine and Chiropractic have so many similarities. Yet and still (pun intended), the degrees conferred by their respective schools are different and the training has several major differences.

THE PHYSIOLOGY OF SPINAL MANIPULATIVE THERAPY

SMT is a therapy that attempts to "adjust" the spine and place it back into proper "alignment." The proper alignment is thought to reduce spinal muscle spasm, joint pain, ligament tension, and tendon tension. The actual maneuvers may cause a "pop" when the spine re-aligns. The "pop" is similar to the sound that is made when someone "cracks their knuckles." A sense of relief is often felt by the patient after the "pop." The person receiving the SMT is usually laying on a special examining table that allows the doctor to have a mechanical advantage for the maneuver. These tables are usually lower and firmer than a conventional examination table.

Secret Number 2: SMT effects the neuro-reflexes of the spine, spinal cord, and brain.

The treatment itself may only take a few seconds. The doctor performing the treatment is required to rotate and bend the patient's spine into what can seem an awkward position. The process requires certain physicality by the performing Doctor. Large patients can prove difficult to align if the Doctor is of a slight build.

The actual mechanism for the "pop" sound and why patients feel relief is not actually known. The sound may be coming from within the small joints of the vertebrae called facet joints. Alternatively, the sound may be generated by the vibration of the small tendons and ligaments of the spine. Each vertebra is surrounded by a network of nerves. When the vertebrae are misaligned (called "subluxations"), the stretch causes stimulation of the nerves and the generation of pain. The thinking is that the realignment removes this tension reducing pain by removing nerve activation.

Furthermore, the nerves that are stretched can cause reflex muscle contraction (spasm) which may be the human body's attempt to realign the spine itself. SMT reduces the muscle spasm by decreasing the nerve activation around the vertebrae. Some patients obtain immediate muscle relaxation after SMT is applied.   Recent studies comparing SMT and other forms of physical therapy have shown symptomatic benefit for the patient. Every year in the U.S. 22 million Americans seek Chiropractic care. About 35% of these cases are for relief of back pain.

SMT INDICATIONS

People seek SMT for the following conditions (see the above diagram):

- Low Back Sprain and Strain
- Neck Sprain and Strain
- Degenerative Disc Disease of the Spine
- Osteoarthritis of the Spine
- Scoliosis
- Headaches

SMT FREQUENCY

The number of treatments and type of SMT is guided by a number of factors such as cause of pain, severity of the pain, and insurance coverage. Generally, people will require more than one or 2 treatments. Multiple treatments over many weeks is the norm (as it would be with physical therapy or therapeutic exercises).

THE RISKS AND SIDE EFFECTS OF SMT

There have been reports of serious spinal injury with SMT. A careful look at those case reports reveals that the Doctor really should have been able to predict that a serious spinal abnormality was present. Most practitioners that utilize SMT today will only apply that form of therapy when the spine has been cleared of any dangerous underlying conditions. Most patients having SMT will have had X-Rays of the spine, a CT scan, or an MRI. When the proper diagnostic workup has been done, SMT is very safe. In fact, if all back therapies were compared, SMT is one of the safest therapies a person with spinal pain can receive.

Secret Number 3: SMT is a safe form of pain management therapy.

Chiropractors practice a very low-risk type of therapy. This is not only evidenced by the extremely low complication rate of SMT but is also evidenced by the cost of malpractice insurance for Chiropractors. Chiropractors pay some of the lowest rates for their malpractice insurance. If their therapies were risky, the insurance companies would charge much higher rates. Most Americans understand how readily an insurance company will raise the cost of coverage for nearly any risk. The low rates reflect their confidence in the safe nature of SMT.

IN CONCLUSION

SMT is an effective form of treatment for certain types of spinal pain. It compares favorably with spinal physical therapy and can be used as an adjunct to a comprehensive spinal program. SMT certainly carries less risk than other more invasive back therapies (such as surgery). It seems to be a reasonable method of therapy to try.

THIS SECTION ON SMT IS FOR INFORMATIONAL USE AND IS NOT INTENDED TO REPLACE THE THOROUGH HISTORY, PHYSICAL, DIAGNOSTIC STUDIES, AND MANAGEMENT BY A LICENSED MEDICAL PRACTITIONER.

VI. Spinal Traction Secrets

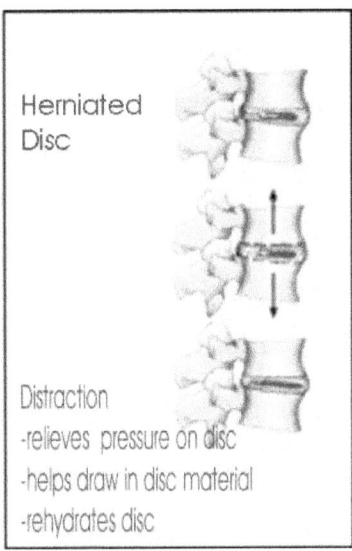

Herniated Disc

Distraction
-relieves pressure on disc
-helps draw in disc material
-rehydrates disc

Although chronic low back pain is frequently alleviated by the previous therapies mentioned many people will require a more intensive form of therapy - low back traction. In the "old days" people were hospitalized, placed on bed rest, and a traction device was attached to the footboard of their bed. Depending on the size of the person, as much as 45 pounds of counterweight connected to a lumbar traction belt would be applied to the person. It was costly, time-consuming, uncomfortable, and didn't work that well. In fact, prospective studies showed that the bed rest alone was as effective as the bed rest with traction.

Secret Number 1: Traction at bed rest does not work that well.

THE PHYSIOLOGIC MECHANSIM OF TRACTION

The concept behind traction is that the lumbar vertebrae are distracted or pulled apart to alleviate the pain (see the above diagram). This stretches the lower back muscles, aligns the spine, pulls the vertebral structures away from compressing the spinal nerves, creates a vacuum within the disc to shrink a herniated disc bulge, and causes the discs to "soak up" fluid thereby expanding the water content of the disc enlarging it.

Secret Number 2: Effective traction can actually improve the structure and function of a disc.

IN CONCLUSION...

In my mind, the best low back traction device would be comfortable, allowing a person to wear it for hours while engaging in light activities. It would also be adjustable as to the amount of abdominal constriction and able to have the traction effect increased or decreased. This would lead to the best low back traction relief of pain. Ideally it would also be easily cleaned and aesthetically pleasing.

Secret Number 3: Portable Traction devices have been shown to be very effective for discogenic disease (especially in the L5 – S1 position).

Sounds like a tall order doesn't it? There actually are several portable devices that are available. In my practice, we used portable traction devices and found them to be very effective (especially for herniation of the L-5 – S-1 disc). I have devoted an entire section later in this book reviewing a particular traction device that has several studies supporting its use. Traction is a very effective form of pain management for people with discogenic pain.

Do not initiate this type of therapy without the approval and supervision by your Doctor.

VII. Joint Injection Therapy Secrets

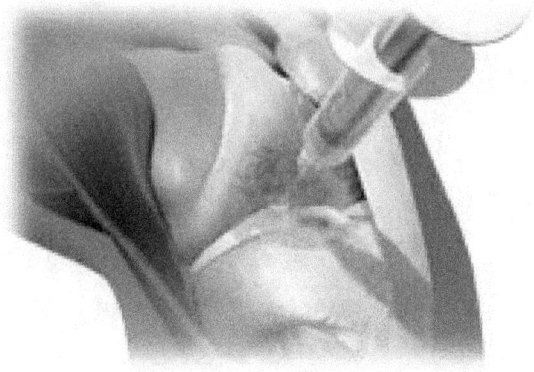

The knee is the most commonly injured joint in people who are physically active. The majority of people who presented themselves for joint injection to my pain practice were people with some type of knee malady. I am going to share my approach to the knee injection technique.

MY HISTORY WITH KNEE INJECTIONS

This is an approach that took me over 20 years to perfect as I performed dozens of knee injections every year in my practice. It is the technique that evolved as I carefully listened to my patients reports of relief (or lack of it), evaluated the medical literature, and pondered the physics of injection technique. I believe you are going to learn some things that you have never heard before (even if you are a healthcare practitioner).

ANATOMY AND PHYSIOLOGY OF THE KNEE

The knee is a mechanically "at risk" joint. What I mean by that is that the very structure of the knee places mechanical forces on it that can amplify "wear and tear." You can think of the mechanical disadvantage of the knee this way...two long poles attached by cords attempting to limit the backward and forward...side to side motion at the ends where the 2 poles meet...that's the knee. When the knee is involved in activity, it moves in a multi-planar way (though its major motion is like a "swinging hinge"). In motion, all attachment and cartilage tissues of the knee are stressed. When standing erect the knee rotates slightly, "locks out," and handles its weight load with a minimum of ligament and tendon strain.

The knee also has two curious interior structures called menisci (meniscus in the singular). The menisci guide the synovial surfaces of the knee and help decrease the "backward and forward – side to side" motion of the knee. They stabilize the sliding surfaces, disperse friction, and cushion the knee. They are made of fibrocartilage (similar to the substance of the outer ring of an intervertebral disc).

Even at bed rest the knee is moving (just ask a friend who has had knee surgery). There is no possible way to eliminate motion of the knee without fusing it. Fusion is a surgical procedure where the femur (upper leg bone) and tibia (lower leg bone) are surgically made into one long pole. Although this may reduce or eliminate knee pain, the additional stress on other joints (namely the hip) often results in earlier hip deterioration necessitating eventual surgery of the hip.

Secret Number 1: The joint of the knee moves even at bed rest.

Even bracing of the knee gives it little support. Orthopedic studies done on football offensive lineman (the largest people in professional American football) show that a knee brace works by reminding the lineman to reduce the strain on their knees by changing the way they block. It offers little measurable supportive help. In my practice, I found bracing good for relief of minor joint pain.

In the standing position, the knee ligaments (which attach one bone to another) and tendons (which attach muscle to bone) are at low stress. The major stress standing is compressive and is applied to the cartilage located on the end of the tibia and femur (called synovial cartilage). As the knee begins to bend, the patellar tendon tension (the patella is the "kneecap") begins to rise first. As motion continues, tension in most ligaments and tendons builds to reach maximum stress at the fully bent position (the "squat"). A full squat places great tension on the majority of the structures of the knee.

Ironically, the knee is the most vulnerable to external forces in its least stressed position, the partially bent knee (5 or 10 degrees of bend). Presumably, this position allows external forces to separate the knee compartments easiest due to relative ligament and tendon laxity. Ligament shearing remains a major mechanism of injury in sports. More recent orthopedic surgical techniques utilizing cadaver ligament and tendon transplants (called allograft transplants), as well as tendon transplants from one part of the same person's body to another (called autograft transplants), have improved recovery from cruciate ligament tears. Ligament looseness (called "laxity"), tendon looseness (also "laxity"), and loss of cartilage of the knee are usual with the aging process. Injury of the knee at an earlier age accelerates the aging process of it. If a human being lives long enough, they will develop some degree of knee problem.

KNEE INJECTION INDICATIONS

The following conditions of the knee have been found to have the chronic pain they cause reduced by knee injections:

- Degenerative Joint Disease of the Knee (this is the most common reason for knee injections).
- Patellar Chondromalacia (a wearing away of the cartilage on the under surface of the kneecap).
- Rheumatoid Arthritis of the Knee
- Other Autoimmune Conditions of the Knee
- Select Ligamentous and Tendinous Conditions of the Knee
- Select Cystic Conditions of the Knee Cartilage
- Select Tumorous Growths of the Knee

THE MEDICATIONS USED FOR KNEE INJECTIONS

The following medications are often used alone or in conjunction with each other when performing a knee injection:

- A local anesthetic agent (such as Lidocaine)
- An injectable corticosteroid (such as cortisone)
- A skin preparatory agent to disinfect the skin prior to injection
- A skin anesthetic agent to reduce the pain of the injection

The medications I used were as follows and for the following reasons:

1) Marcaine 0.25% solution in a multi-dose vial:

I liked this long-acting local anesthetic agent because it gave fairly rapid pain relief (within minutes) and persisted until the other medicines in the "mix" could begin to work. *If you look at the literature about this anesthetic agent it is not officially approved for joint injections.* This is because it can cause cartilage damage when used as a continuous infusion into the joint (such as after surgery) when using the 0.5% concentration. In my mix, I used the 0.25% solution and never more than 1cc (mixed with 2 ccs of other fluids). This very low concentration of Marcaine never caused any reactions in any patients in over 26 years of practice.

2) Depo-Medrol 40 mg per cc multi-dose vial:

This is a moderate acting corticosteroid in a suspension (there are tiny micro-particles of steroid) which prolongs the duration of action of the medicine. Although there are many side effects that can occur with the systemic administration of corticosteroids, when given into a joint the systemic absorption is much less and subsequently the side effects are less also. This substance is anti-inflammatory and will "calm down" the swelling that can occur in certain knee conditions. My dose was 1 cc (or 40 mg) mixed with 1 cc of Marcaine and another 1 cc of a substance called Sarapin.

3) Sarapin is a natural anti-inflammatory made from the Pitcher plant.

I used a multi-dose vial of this substance and added 1 cc of it to my injectable mix. It has no side effects and never provoked any reactions in over 26 years of giving joint injections.

THEREFORE, THE INJECTABLE MIX THAT I USED IN MY PAIN MANAGEMENT PRACTICE FOR OVER 26 YEARS WAS A MIXTURE OF 1 CC OF MARCAINE 0.25 % TO 1 CC OF DEPOMEDROL 40 MG PER CC TO 1 CC OF SARAPIN. THE TOTAL VOLUME FOR THE KNEE INJECTION WAS 3 CC.

Secret Number 2: Limiting the concentration and strength of the medications used in a knee injection allows the knee to be injected more frequently without diminishing the pain relieving effect of the injection.

I believe that the combination of local anesthetic (giving immediate relief) with two anti-inflammatories (the Sarapin diluting and amplifying the Depo-Medrol) was the reason why we had such profoundly positive results with our knee injections. I cannot recall any patient not obtaining relief with our injection mix nor do I recall any serious side effects in nearly 3 decades of performing this type of injection.

THE EQUIPMENT USED IN THE INJECTION

We also used carefully selected equipment when we performed knee injections. Over the years, I noticed that physicians who performed this type of injection were accustomed to using a fairly heavy 18 or 20 gauge needle. The patients would often complain about their past experience with knee injections that, although they obtained some relief, the actual needle insertion was excruciating. This caused them to resist repeat knee injections.

I decided to use a 27-gauge Titanium needle for knee injections (a much thinner needle). The gauge of the needle affects how much pain occurs with the needle stick. Most thin needles are short as they tend to bend easily when thin. The needle for knee injection must be long enough to traverse the centimeter or two of tissue that must be penetrated to enter the joint space of the knee. However, Titanium is a stronger metal and does not bend so easily even when very thin.

I was able to find 1.5-inch Titanium needles that could easily traverse the distance from the skin surface to the interior of the knee. As long as I did not have to remove fluid from the knee (a fluid that is usually like pancake syrup) I could use the thinner needle for injection only. If fluid had to be removed, I would have to resort to the thicker (more painful) 18-gauge needle as you cannot pull out thick fluid with a 27 G needle.

Secret Number 3: The type of equipment used in the knee injection can reduce the pain of the procedure.

I also used 3 cc syringes (sterile single use). The smaller syringe slowed down the velocity of the medicine exiting the needle also reducing the pain evoked by the injection. Every knee injection was done under sterile technique. I always wore sterile, single use gloves and prepped the area with alcohol prior to the injection. When prepping we always waited until the disinfectant dried as it is only effective having dried. In my training I recall many Doctors injecting before the skin prep had dried. I believe our habit of waiting a few extra minutes until drying occurred may be the reason why there was never an injection-related infection in nearly 27 years of doing these injections.

THE INJECTION TECHNIQUE

There are several approaches to inserting the needle. In my training, I was taught to lay the patient down and, while their leg was straight at the knee, slide the needle under the knee cap (the patella) from the side to enter the interior of the knee for injection. Many patients found this rather uncomfortable as perhaps 50% of the time the

Doctor will find themselves scraping the bottom of the patella as the needle is advanced. This can cause severe pain.

Alternatively, I changed my approach and had the patient sit on the end of the examining table with the knee bent at 90 degrees. In this position, the patella "hugs" the femur and 2 very ample spaces open on either side of it (see the above diagram). The needle is then passed a short distance through the skin where it can then enter the interior of the knee without scraping any bone surfaces or cartilage. Overall, my patients told me it was the most painless knee injection they ever had. They would return without any pre-injection anxiety when the previous injections had been nearly painless.

THE SIDE EFFECTS OF KNEE INJECTION

As I have already stated, I cannot recall any side effects, allergic reactions, or infections that resulted from injections of the knee. Naturally, any allergic history the patient may have regarding the substances used for this procedure must be identified before the injection. I would never inject an already infected knee (drainage only).   Furthermore, I always avoided puncturing the skin if there was evidence of infection at the puncture site or a large varicose vein. To me, these are common sense and may not even be worthy of mentioning. Every one of my patients, and I mean everyone, received significant relief from our knee injection technique. I always made sure that we had an accurate diagnosis prior to the procedure and never injected someone with an acute knee injury.

THE FREQUENCY OF KNEE INJECTION

The Orthopedic literature on knee injections all seems to limit the number of injections to no more than four per year. If you examine those studies done, they are fairly poorly structured. Sometimes in medicine a certain habit gets taught and ingrained into Doctors without it really being the truth. Because of this I believe that knee injections can be safely given more frequently than the time held tradition of no more than four per year.

The challenge my patients had was that their pain returned a few weeks after their injection. What were they to do if their next injection was two or three months away? This also prompted me to lighten the doses of each injectable (as I have already enumerated) so that I could increase the frequency of injection. *I would estimate that, in my practice, the average patient who was on a knee injection schedule came in every 4 weeks.*

IN CONCLUSION

WITH THE TECHNIQUE I HAVE DESCRIBED MY PATIENTS ALWAYS RECEIVED A REDUCTION IN THEIR PAIN, THERE

WERE NEVER ANY REPORTED SIDE EFFECTS, NEVER ANY REPORTED ALLERGIC REACTIONS, AND NEVER ANY INJECTION ASSOCIATED INFECTIONS. ON AVERAGE, I SAW TWO OR THREE PEOPLE PER WEEK FOR KNEE INJECTIONS FOR OVER 26 YEARS. SURELY THIS IS LONG ENOUGH TO OBSERVE ANY ILL EFFECTS THAT MAY HAVE OCCURRED FROM OUR INJECTION TECHNIQUE.

THIS CHAPTER IS INTENDED AS INFORMATIONAL ONLY. EVERY PATIENT RECEIVING A KNEE INJECTION MUST HAVE A THOROUGH HISTORY AND PHYSICAL PERFORMED BY A LICENSED MEDICAL PRACTITIONER AND HAVE THEIR INJECTIONS DONE BY TRAINED PERSONNEL.

I have carefully enumerated my way to perform a knee injection. You now know more about the technique than most physicians do. I would recommend you find a practitioner who is willing to do your knee injection by the technique I have just taught you. You will find it to be nearly painless, have few side effects, and it will be very effective at relieving your pain.

VIII. Spinal Injection Therapy Secrets

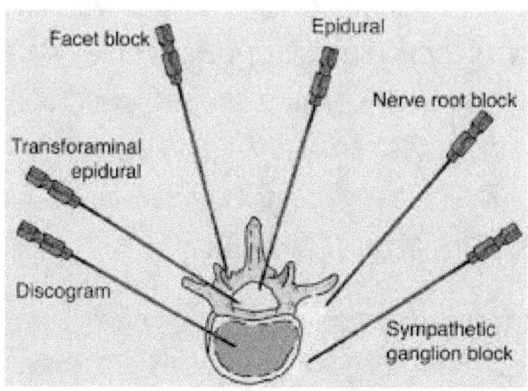

With an estimated 100 million Americans suffering from chronic pain, relief of pain seems to be more elusive than ever. Surely, spinal injections for back pain are better than using opiate pain medications, right? Not necessarily. There were 8.9 million Americans who received injections for pain last year. Just how effective were those injections for relief of pain? This section is going to review spinal injection for back pain as an alternative to other modalities for pain relief. The choice to have one of these types of injections is complicated.

GENERAL CONSIDERATIONS ABOUT SPINAL INJECTIONS

Deciding to have spinal injections is a complicated menagerie of what injection might work (there is no perfect way to know beforehand), what the patient can tolerate, what the Doctor thinks is indicated, and what your insurance will pay. Furthermore, there needs to be an access to an accredited facility where the Doctors perform them. Most patients will require multiple injections and will receive temporary relief. If the patient's pain worsens in-between injections, they will usually have to wait for their next scheduled session.

Secret Number 1: The effectiveness of spinal injections for chronic back pain is limited.

Generally, insurance companies will limit the number and frequency of injections they will pay for. The administering physician will try to select the most effective injection techniques for the patient (the acceptable effectiveness is only a 30% reduction in pain). *The Food and Drug Administration has never endorsed steroid spinal injections.* Those types of injections occupy a "gray area" in the field of pain management called "off-label usage." Many things in medicine actually fall into this category because scientific studies for effectiveness are difficult to fund, perform, and structure.

Many authorities in pain management feel very ambivalent about spinal injections for chronic back pain. The effectiveness for acute lumbar disc herniation is much clearer. As the pain becomes more chronic the effectiveness of injection therapies becomes less obvious. So spinal injection therapy is really an attempt to find an effective alternative to having to use other expensive, chronic therapies (that also have a lukewarm effectiveness in treating chronic pain). As it turns out, there is no injection therapy available for chronic pain which is not costly and risky.

Secret Number 2: There is no way to definitively predict, before the injection, which spinal injection will work best for chronic low back pain (as there are usually multiple mechanisms for the pain).

TYPES OF SPINAL INJECTIONS

There are three basic types of spinal injections:

1) Intervertebral Epidural Injections: in this type of injection a small volume of medicine is injected into a space around the spinal cord called the epidural space. The medicine injected will numb the nerves and decrease the swelling that is pushing against the nerves in the lower back. This is a sterile procedure and is best done with the patient lightly anesthetized (similar to the anesthesia for a colonoscopy). Sometimes the Doctor performing the procedure will use X-Ray techniques during the procedure to ensure better needle placement.

2) Facet or Foramina Injections: in this type of injection a very small volume of medicine (similar in type but a smaller amount than used in an epidural) is injected into or near a joint or nerve foramen on the vertebrae. Using

X-Ray guidance is the best way to do this type of injection as the area being injected is very small.

3) Caudal Epidural Injection: this is a type of epidural injection that is given very low on the spine in an area called the sacral hiatus. It is useful for very low disc herniation (Lumbar 5 for instance) and can be done without anesthesia with just sterile draping and instruments.

Though there are many other types of injections and variations, the above 3 constitute the most frequently employed techniques. They require a minimum of surgical skill and have minimal risk of complications.

INDICATIONS FOR A SPINAL INJECTION

The potential disorders that may be treated by these types of procedures are as follows:

- Non-fragmented Herniated Disc of the Spine
- Degenerative Joint Disease
- Degenerative Disc Disease
- Spinal Stenosis
- Scoliosis
- Spinal Neuropathic Pain
- Spinal Trauma
- "Failed Back Syndrome" (chronic low back pain after multiple back surgeries)

- Compression Fractures
- Synovial Cyst
- Arthritic Syndromes of the back
- Disc Bulge
- Disc Tear

This is not an exhaustive list of indications but includes most of the reasons an injection would be done.

The administration of a spinal injection for back pain is not usually performed by a primary care practitioner. Usually, the patient will need referral to a specialist that is trained in the technique. In all cases, an MRI of the spine (with contrast) will need to be performed before a thorough recommendation can be made. I recommend that the injections be performed under anesthesia when there is no reason to not do so. Since the procedure will likely have to be repeated, making the experience as pleasant as possible for the patient is wisdom. Furthermore, optimal positioning for the procedure is easier under anesthesia (pain in an awake patient will often limit positioning).

Secret Number 3: The skill of the professional performing the injection correlates highly with its effectiveness for relief of pain. There is currently no registry of spinal injecting physicians that evaluates their skill so that a patient can make an informed decision.

CONDITIONS WHERE THE RISK OF SPINAL INJECTION OUTWEIGHS THE BENEFIT

The following conditions make the administering of a spinal injection too high a risk and should not be performed:

- Blood clotting problems
- Infection
- Breathing Problems
- Unstable physiology (such as a person with serious heart disease)
- Allergy to any of the medicines used in the procedure
- Adamant refusal by the patient
- Untrained person attempting to do the procedure
- Improper sterile technique
- Insufficient equipment
- Inability to effectively resuscitate the patient in the event of an emergency (that means the right equipment and trained personnel must be present).
- Brain Tumor
- Spinal Cord Tumor
- Meningitis
- Encephalitis
- Hydrocephalus
- Morbid Obesity

The conditions mentioned above are not an exhaustive list but constitute the majority of reasons that a spinal injection should not be done.

IN CONCLUSION

I have reviewed for you the major spinal injections for back pain, the indications, the process of setting up an injection, and the reasons to not have an injection done. These injections are considered "safe" but no injection or surgical procedure is without potential side effects and complications. This therapy should only follow a thorough history, physical, MRI, and evaluation by a licensed medical practitioner. The medical professional performing the procedure should be trained in all aspects of this technique.

The usefulness of these injection techniques for chronic back pain is very limited. If after one or two injection sessions the pain recurs shortly afterward, the likelihood for prolonged relief is very low. It is my opinion that this form of therapy is not as reliable a way to reduce chronic back pain as several other therapies in this book.

IX. Back Bracing Therapy Secrets

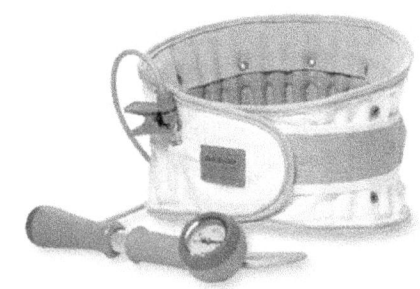

Many people with chronic lumbar (lower back) pain will want to consider the use of a lumbar back brace. If you have had any experience in trying to find the right type of brace, then you know it can be daunting. It has been estimated that 31 million Americans suffer from chronic lumbar pain...you are not alone in your dilemma.

You would be amazed at the number of people who suffer from chronic lumbar pain who have not been given an actual diagnosis   Before attempting bracing therapy you should have had a complete history and physical, an MRI of your lumbar spine, and had a trial of treatment by a team of pain practitioners (Physical Therapist, Orthopedic Surgeon, etc.). If this has not been done, you need to see your primary care practitioner BEFORE you go any further in your search for a brace.

Secret Number 1: Back bracing works best when it is part of a comprehensive back rehabilitation program.

If you are hoping to reduce your chronic lumbar pain with the brace alone, you are going to be disappointed. The causes of chronic low back pain are many and often a person has two or more overlapping neuro-mechanisms. So...a back brace should be only one component of a regimen of exercise, medications, physical therapy, etc. Your primary care practitioner should be able to construct this regimen for you.

THE NEURO-MECHANISM FOR PAIN RELIEF WITH BRACING

The ways in which bracing relieves pain can be summarized by 6 separate neuro-mechanisms:

1. *Alignment:* Each segment of your spine moves in multiple directions. Over time segments of your spine "get stuck" which can stretch nerves, muscles, ligaments, tendons, joint capsules, etc. This causes pain and is relieved when the brace coaxes your spine back into alignment.
2. *Supportive:* Gravity is constantly stressing your spine. The nerves, ligaments, tendons, and discs are designed to be the supportive network for your

spine. A lumbar brace compresses your abdominal contents causing a supportive effect on your spine.

3. *Restrictive:* A brace decreases the range of motion of your spine, thus decreasing pain. Recent studies have shown that bracing causes a person to unconsciously reduce their range of motion (admittedly there is a small number of people who actually do the opposite and cause further damage).

4. *Traction:* There are several braces on the market that actually apply traction to the lumbar spine relieving some of the compressive effects of gravity (see the above diagram).

5. *Psychosomatic Effect:* There is a sense of security some people get when they wear a brace. This can actually cause the release of endorphins in the brain which are naturally occurring pain relievers.

6. *Direct Contact Therapies*: Several types of lumbar braces have devices embedded in their structure which can have therapeutic effects on pain (for instance some braces have hot packs or magnets in them).

Secret Number 2: Back bracing works best when the brace is selected based on the mechanism generating the low back pain.

TYPES OF BRACES

There are a range of types of lumbar back braces. A back brace may offer Support, Compression of the Abdomen, Restriction, or Traction. Many lumbar back braces offer combinations of these types in a single brace. In particular, the traction braces are well suited to relieve chronic lumbar spinal pain from spinal nerve compression due to disc herniation.

FITTING THE BRACE

When fitting your back brace, you will want it snug but not restricting breathing. You should be able to slide your little finger along the side of the brace between your skin and the brace. Also take note whether you will be wearing the brace directly against the skin or not. If against the skin you will want to see if you are allergic to the contact material the brace is made from.

Secret Number 3: Back braces are not intended to be worn 24 hours a day.

DURATION OF WEARING THE BRACE

Most health care practitioners do not recommend continuous wearing of your lumbar brace. You may only need to wear the brace when you are active, or working, or have persistent pain.

Remember that your brace is not a replacement for a good history and physical by your primary care practitioner. You will want to coordinate the type of brace you select with your practitioner.

IN CONCLUSION

I hope this section has given you some additional guidance on how to select a lumbar back brace. You will find that the proper brace for you is a very individualized choice. When you find the right brace, you will have less pain, more liberty to do things, and more independence.

X. Massage Therapy Secrets

Do you suffer from muscular discomfort, tension, aches, or a sports injury?

Sports Injury (Upper & Lower Body)

Headaches & Migraine

Neck Ache, Whiplash

Shoulder Problems

Ligament & Tendon Problems (Upper & Lower Body)

Muscle Stiffness, Aches & Tension (Upper & Lower Body)

Tennis Elbow

Lower Back Problems

RSI, Carpal Tunnel

Hip, Pelvis & Leg Discomfort

Massage can help you feel human again.

Who doesn't like Massage Therapy (MT)? In 2007, the American Massage Therapy Association noted in a survey that nearly 25% of all adult Americans had MT at least once in the previous year. So that means about 80 million Americans had MT in 2006. Could they all have been misled to MT's benefits? I doubt it. However, what are the massage therapy facts? What is it, how does it work, and what is it good for? Could there be times when you shouldn't have MT? Let's see if I can answer those questions in this section.

Secret Number 1: The style of Massage Therapy is individualized to each condition and objective for the therapy.

TYPES OF MASSAGE THERAPY

There are over 80 different MT styles. Each style has variations in pressure, movements, and techniques. Also, different areas of the body can be the focus of MT. In some cases, a total body massage is preferred (such as when the purpose is to evoke total body relaxation). There are also times when only one area of the body is the focus (such as in headache relief). The decision as to what type is best for you depends on your preferences, your massage therapist's recommendation, and the particular relief you are looking for.

THE PHYSIOLOGY OF MASSAGE THERAPY

Secret Number 2: Massage Therapy has 4 different mechanisms through which it relieves pain.

MT works through several different physiological mechanisms (physiology is the study of how the body works). The major mechanisms are as follows:

- *"Counter-irritation"*: Any stimulus of the skin surface causes reactivity in the spinal cord. Different types of stimuli affect the spinal cord in different ways. From rubbing the skin to deep pressure over "trigger points" (focal areas of pain), a "Gating Mechanism" in the spinal cord can be activated. Drs. Melzack and Wall described the "Gate Theory" of pain transmission in the spinal cord in 1965. They hypothesized that the transmission of pain works like a gate. If the gate is open, the pain is transmitted to the brain and perceived. Conversely, if the gate is closed (by a "counter-irritation" stimulus), the pain signal does not transmit up the spinal cord. Most of the pain therapies that are applied to the skin work by this mechanism.
- *Resetting of Muscle Tension:* the given resting tone of muscle is called "muscle tension." It is neurologically preset by receptors in the muscle.

By resetting the resting tension, one can achieve relaxation of the targeted muscle. When a muscle or group of muscles are stretched it can reset the resting tension. Muscle with a high resting tension require more nutrients. The result can be pain and fatigue. MT is excellent for resetting resting muscle tension.

- *Improvement of Blood and Tissue Fluid Flow*: by compressing and releasing areas with MT the dynamics of the fluids which carry nutrients to and waste products away from body tissues is affected. This is a "hydraulic pumping effect" as well as "syphoning effect" with MT. The net result is to improve nutrient flow and remove the metabolic waste products that accumulate in damaged tissue. Healing can be enhanced and further damage reduced.

- *Neuro-transmitter Release:* the stimulation of the aforementioned processes also results in the release of chemical substances that mediate pain perception. These substances are called "Neuro-transmitters." They are the chemical substances of the nervous system that "fine tune" the electrical signaling in the nervous system. The names of these substances are many. Endorphins, Serotonin, Dopamine, Oxytocin, and a host of others are all positively affected by MT. Our understanding of what these substances do seems to be constantly growing. New transmitters are regularly discovered. Not only do these substances affect your perception of pain but also affect your sense of well-being. Anxiety, Depression, and Post Traumatic Stress Disorder are all related to negative fluctuations of these neuro-chemicals.

INDICATIONS FOR MASSAGE THERAPY

The following conditions have been shown to have pain reduction with MT (see the above diagram):

- Chronic Headaches
- Whiplash
- Chronic Neck Pain
- Chronic Back Pain
- Chronic Joint Pain
- Pain from prolonged bed rest
- Fibromyalgia
- Chronic Fatigue Syndrome
- Chronic Shoulder Pain
- TMJ
- RSD
- Carpal Tunnel Syndrome
- Multiple Sclerosis
- Spinal Cord Injuries

Of course, this is not a complete listing.

PRECAUTIONS WITH MASSAGE THERAPY

Secret Number 3: Massage Therapy is not indicated in conditions where a clot could be dislodged.

MT is a very safe form of therapy for relief for chronic pain.   The following may be situations where MT is ill-advised:

- *Conditions where the presence of an underlying blood clot is possible.* Massage of a limb with a blood clot present in the deep venous system could potentially dislodge the clot with serious consequences.

- *Conditions where the pain has not been properly diagnosed.* MT to a fractured spine could result in additional injury. Therefore, it is essential that the cause for your pain to have been thoroughly investigated by a licensed medical practitioner before receiving MT.

- *Conditions where injury can occur with the pressure exerted in MT.* There are both congenital (conditions a person is born with) and acquired (conditions that can develop from certain diseases) where the body is extremely fragile. MT must be very carefully used in these situations.

- *Conditions, where a licensed medical practitioner or massage therapist have advised you, to not have MT.* Think of your massage therapist as another valuable health practitioner...heed their advice.

IN CONCLUSION...

I have reviewed what MT is, how it works, what it is good for, and precautions. The usual challenge a person with chronic pain has with MT is that many medical insurance companies will not cover the cost for it. Before you schedule your appointment with a massage therapist you should check your insurance coverage for it. The coverage varies from state to state and country to country. There is great hope for relief with the application of MT in many conditions.

XI. Acupuncture Secrets

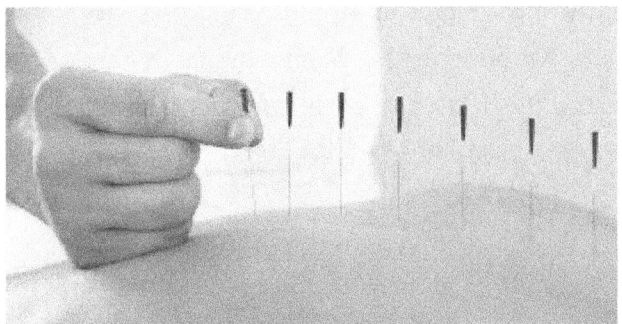

The introduction of Acupuncture as a popular treatment in America for chronic pain really began during the Nixon presidency when China and the United States re-invigorated their trade relations. Since that time, there has been a growing integration of this ancient healing art into mainstream Western medicine. The actual person who invented Acupuncture is unknown. Even the exact time period of its invention is a mystery. What is known is that millions of Chinese people have used it as medical therapy for many centuries.

Secret Number 1: Objective analysis of the benefits of Acupuncture for chronic pain gives mixed results.

The Cochran Review (an organization that evaluates the effectiveness of therapies scientifically) rates the objective information for Acupuncture's effectiveness with mixed results. There are some scientific studies that show benefit while others show it equal to a placebo effect. Presently, most states in the U.S. require licensing for non-physician Acupuncturists. Many physicians have integrated this form of therapy into their practices (especially those physicians who are focused on treating chronic pain).

THE PHYSIOLOGY OF ACUPUNCTURE

There are few good scientific studies for how Acupuncture works. The ancient Chinese explanation revolves around the concept of body energy (called Chi). The Chinese believed that by placing needles into various points in the body (called meridians) you could "balance" the Chi. They believed that an imbalance of the Chi causes illness. Curiously, the meridians on ancient Chinese charts mirror the locations where a specialized type of nerve fiber (called a C nerve fiber) can be found anatomically. C fibers are slow conducting nerve fibers that transmit chronic pain signals.

Secret Number 2: Acupuncture probably works through a "Gating Mechanism" in the spinal cord to close pain transmission.

Acute pain is transmitted by a different type of nerve fiber called an A-delta fiber. These types of fibers are very rapid conducting. Their pathways do not correspond to the ancient Chinese meridians. Much of what I am telling you is fairly recent neuroscience information. The C-fiber arrangement varies from one person to the next. They are also very tiny and difficult to identify on gross anatomy dissection. The C-fiber pattern variation from person to person may help explain why there can be great variability in the effectiveness of Acupuncture from person to person.

By stimulating the C-fibers that are connected to a particular organ system a "counter-irritative" stimulus travels to the spinal cord and "closes the gate" on pain transmission. The "Gate Theory" of pain transmission was originally described by Drs. Melzack and Wall in 1965. Once the Acupuncture needles are placed in their appropriate meridian, they can be spun, heated, an electrical stimulus applied, or a laser applied. The very fact that a needle is inserted serves as a "counter-irritative" stimulus. Though this may seem strange to you, the same mechanism is in play when you get a massage, or apply a pain relieving cream, or even a TENS unit. Any irritative stimulus applied to the skin can have a "Gating Effect."

ACUPUNCTURE INDICATIONS

The following conditions have been shown to be effectively treated with Acupuncture:

- Chemotherapy-induced vomiting
- After surgery vomiting
- Dental pain
- Fibromyalgia
- Labor pain

- Chronic neck pain
- Chronic low back pain
- Headaches
- Osteoarthritis
- Menstrual Cramps

There may be other conditions that can be treated, but the ones I have listed show the most consistent support in the medical literature.

ACUPUNCTURE PRECAUTIONS

Secret Number 3: Acupuncture should not be used in pregnant women.

Generally, Acupuncture is safe. In the following conditions Acupuncture is to be avoided:

- People with bleeding tendencies. That includes people who are on "blood thinners" for certain medical conditions.
- Pregnant women as Acupuncture may induce labor.
- People with an implanted electrical device (such as a pacemaker) as the electrical stimulus applied to Acupuncture needles could cause the device to malfunction.

There are few complications that can occur with receiving Acupuncture. The most common (and avoidable) complication is an infection. The needles used should be sterile and the skin should be prepped with alcohol or some other solution before insertion. These simple measures should avoid any significant infectious complications.

SIDE EFFECTS OF ACUPUNCTURE

- There have been several reports of organ puncture with deep needle insertion. I would imagine that this complication is more likely in a very thin person. A trained, competent, responsible Acupuncturist will be able to avoid this complication.
- One should expect some soreness after an Acupuncture treatment. After all, your skin has been pierced. This should be short lived and quite minor (as the needles are so thin).
- There may be a small amount of pain with needle insertion. Needle pain is largely due to the thickness of a needle, the sharpness of the needle (dull needles hurt more), the area being pierced, the length of the needle, the pain threshold of the person receiving the needle puncture, and the irritative effects of what may

be attached to the needle. Acupuncture needle insertion is nearly painless.

IN CONCLUSION

Many insurance companies do not cover Acupuncture. Be sure to check with your particular insurance carrier before scheduling your appointment. A licensed Acupuncturist or Physician is best for this type of therapy. You can expect your appointment and therapy to last no more than an hour. You will probably be invited for treatments once or twice a week for several weeks. Acupuncture treatments usually take several sessions to see results. Overall this type of therapy offers hope for relief of many forms of chronic pain.

XII. Spinal Surgery Secrets

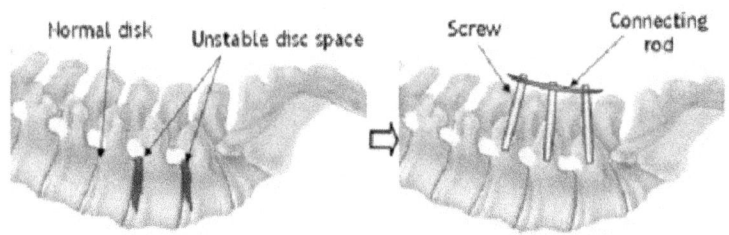

(a) Before fusion.   (b) After fusion.

A method of the spinal fusion surgery

254 | P a g e

To date, there have been no reliable studies that recommend lower lumbar surgery for chronic back pain. The surgical literature is clear on acute low back pain and the benefit of surgery when the workup reveals a problem that can be treated surgically (such as disc material extruding into the spinal canal). Many people with chronic back pain have two or more neuro-mechanisms for their pain. When there are several overlapping mechanisms for the pain (a mechanism is how the pain is actually being generated) surgery for chronic low back pain has not been proven to be more effective than other less invasive forms of therapy (such as therapeutic exercise).

Secret Number 1: Surgery has never been proven to be better for chronic low back pain than other less invasive therapies.

THE PRE-SURGICAL WORKUP

If you have chronic back pain (pain that is continuous for three months or more) and you are contemplating surgery you should have accomplished the following things:

- *You should have had a thorough history and physical by a licensed medical practitioner who is experienced in chronic lumbar pain.*

- *You should have had a lumbar MRI with contrast to evaluate for the anatomical possibilities of the neuro-mechanism for the pain.*
- *You should have failed a trial of less invasive therapy that was prescribed by a team of experts (Rehabilitation Specialist, Spinal Orthopedic or Neurosurgeon, Pain Specialist).*
- *You will need to get at least two opinions from Surgical Specialists that sub-specialize in lower lumbar surgery (usually an Orthopedic Surgeon or a Neurosurgeon). Each opinion should agree that surgery is your best option.*

Secret Number 2: A surgical cure for chronic low back pain should only be considered after other non-invasive therapies have been attempted.

IN CONCLUSION

It will take a little courage on your part, but you should check on the surgeon's credentials, in what hospital the surgery will be performed, and how many lumbar operations the surgeon does per year (it should be more than 25). Of course, there are no guarantees with any surgery. You cannot eliminate complications...only reduce them. Remember, several million Americans undergo surgery each year without any serious complications. Follow these basic guidelines to have the best outcome possible.

Often an intensive trial of traction therapy will result in enough pain relief that surgery is not necessary. This option must be reviewed with your supervising medical practitioner.

Secret Number 3: A surgical cure for chronic low back pain should only be performed by an Orthopedic Surgeon, who sub-specializes in spinal surgery.

THIS CHAPTER IS NOT INTENDED AS MEDICAL ADVICE BUT INFORMATIONAL ONLY. IF YOU INTEND TO PURSUE SURGERY YOU SHOULD DO SO UNDER THE SUPERVISION OF A LICENSED MEDICAL PRACTITIONER.

Chapter 9 – Secrets of Uncommon Treatments for Chronic Pain

I. Vitamin D Supplementation Secrets

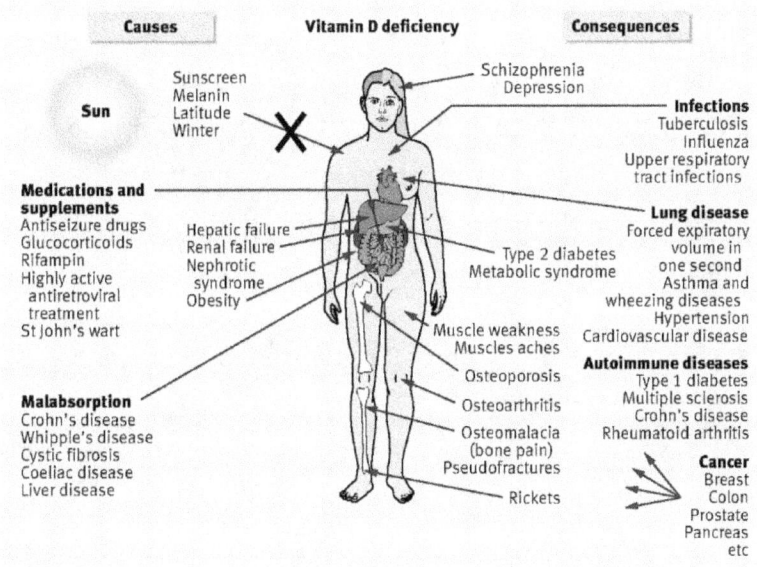

With all the information and disinformation on the internet about nutraceuticals, Vitamin D is a vitamin that you do not want to miss as a supplement to treat chronic pain. The fact is, especially if you live in the northern part of the U.S., you are likely to be Vitamin D deficient during the winter months' even if your diet is adequate (the majority of our Vitamin D is manufactured by skin conversion from sun exposure).

THE PHYSIOLOGY OF VITAMIN D

Vitamin D works by affecting calcium and phosphorus absorption and excretion. It is essential for bone health and has effects on our kidneys, liver, skin, immune system, and central nervous system. In some ways Vitamin D is more a hormone as we don't really need to get it from our diet when we have adequate sun exposure (vitamins are, by definition, coenzymes that our body cannot manufacture). Because Vitamin D has so many effects on the human body, treatment guidelines have been published on the various types of disorders Vitamin D can treat.

Secret Number 1: Vitamin D is a hormone that can be supplemented daily.

CONDITIONS FOR VITAMIN D SUPPLEMENTATION (SEE THE ABOVE DIAGRAM)

The following is a listing of disorders for treatment with Vitamin D:

Vitamin D Supplementation Provides Definite Benefit

- "Rickets" (Vitamin D Deficiency)
- Osteoporosis
- Osteomalacia
- Psoriasis

- Hyperparathyroidism
- Hypoparathyroidism
- Renal Osteodystrophy

Vitamin D Supplementation Has Probable Benefit

- Preventing Falls in the Elderly
- Obesity
- Vascular Disease

Vitamin D Supplementation Has Possible Benefit

- Depression
- Pre-menstrual Syndrome
- Cancer
- Multiple Sclerosis
- Respiratory Infections in Children (Common cold/Influenza)
- Teeth/Gum Disease
- Scleroderma
- Systemic Lupus Erythematosus
- Rheumatoid Arthritis

Secret Number 2: Vitamin D supplementation is essential for maximal health in most adults.

VITAMIN D DOSING GUIDELINES

Vitamin D being a "fat soluble" vitamin can accumulate in your body and cause toxic side effects. When it comes to fat soluble vitamins more is not always better. The dosing range of 400 IU per day to 4000 IU per day has been safely recommended in adults. Because Vitamin D is really a hormone you are taking, consider taking the higher dosage range under the direction of your primary care provider. They may want to check a 25-hydroxyvitamin D level prior to initiating therapy. People who are taking medications that up-regulate liver function (such as medications for epilepsy) may need 2 or 3 times the dose of other people. Finally, people who are taking Diuretics, Calcium Channel Blockers, and Digoxin will want to be guided by their primary care provider also.

Secret Number 3: Checking a 25-hydroxyvitamin D level helps to gauge the daily dose.

IN CONCLUSION

Vitamin D is an essential, inexpensive, and safe supplement that has demonstrated excellent results with pain reduction, enhancing bone health, and treating a wide variety of disorders. This is one supplement that all chronic pain patients will want to consider.

II. Cognitive Behavioral Therapy Secrets

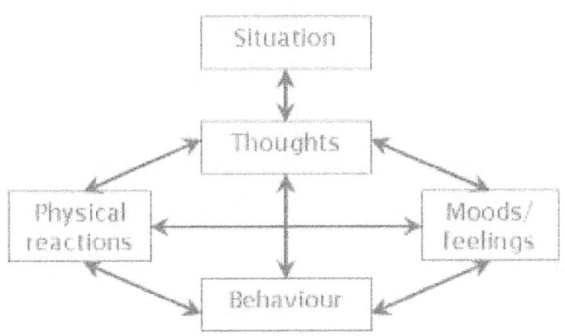

As the field of Neuroscience begins to unravel the intricacies of central nervous pain modulation, the hope for definitive therapies modulating pain at the central nervous system level begin to appear. Cognitive Behavioral Therapy (CBT) is a form of psychotherapy that has been shown to be effective in reducing many forms of pain (as well as several psychiatric disorders). Originally created by Drs. Beck and Ellis, the premise is that maladaptive conditions contribute to emotional distress and the maintenance of behavioral problems. In that anxiety, depression, and insomnia significantly amplify the perception of chronic pain, CBT is a logical adjunct to any chronic pain regimen.

Secret Number 1: CBT should be an adjunct in most people with chronic pain.

THE NEUROPHYSIOLOGY OF CBT

Although the brain has certain modularity (for instance, vision is processed by the occipital lobe of the cortex-located in the back of the brain), the brain is really a vast, interconnected network. There is an emotional response to nearly every conscious function of the brain. The limbic system (located in the center of the brain) acts as a neural intermediary for our brain network and reliably connects an emotional experience to every conscious event (and some unconscious...such as dreaming while asleep).

Even certain unconscious functions can evoke the Limbic system as the neural signaling traverses the brain from one region to the other. The notion that the human brain is only used 10% of the time is a drastic misrepresentation of the truth. Indeed, the brain is never inactive and is networked at all times. Both internal and external stimuli cause the brain to respond. Repeated stimulation of pain pathways causes them to change in structure and function (yes, chronic pain actually changes the anatomy of the brain). Repeated stimulation causes "wind up" which increases the efficiency of pain transmission.

Secret Number 2: CBT causes positive changes in the structure and function of the brain.

With this increase in function, the same pain stimulus causes more pain over time. Pain patients often report worsening of their pain despite there not being any worsening of their disease that is demonstrable with diagnostic studies (such as an MRI). These patients are often accused of simply wanting more pain medication or of being addicts. The automatic neural signaling of the brain is significantly affected by the frontal cortex of the brain (the area for thought – a particularly unique quality of being human). The frontal cortex exerts its influence over many automatic functions of the brain. Because of this, the thoughts and imagination of a person can affect the function of the brain and change it.

The entire process we are talking about is called, "neuroplasticity." The thoughts of a human being actually change the structure and the function of the brain. Consider identical twins...a misnomer really. You see identical twins do not have identical neural networks because their different life experiences modify their neural signaling. There are never two identical people for that reason...ever.

It stands to reason that CBT could influence the processing of pain signaling since CBT affects how one thinks. Recent Neuroscience studies have disclosed that the chemical substances used for one nerve cell to "speak" to another, called neurotransmitters, are actually changed by CBT.

Serotonin, Norepinephrine, Dopamine, and many other neurotransmitters can actually be raised or lowered through CBT. The CBT exerts its effect through frontal lobe activation (remember this is where thought occurs) and modifies the effect of the neurotransmitter. Do this enough and permanent changes occur in the anatomy and physiology of the brain.

This process can be more precise than using medications, electrical stimulation, or surgery as the exact pathways for the chronic pain are being affected. Furthermore, the unique "connectome" or neural network that has been established through years of experiences is precisely affected by CBT. With continued CBT, the "neuroplasticity" that occurs (it generally takes six weeks for this to begin to happen) will result in a significant clinical improvement. Most patients report a reduction in pain, anxiety, insomnia, and depression. Many patients end up taking less medication (and some even wean off their medications).

INDICATIONS FOR CBT

The following disorders have been shown to be improved with CBT:

- Nearly all forms and types of chronic pain
- Fibromyalgia

- Chronic Fatigue
- Chronic Anxiety
- Chronic Depression

In addition to the above disorders, CBT has also shown great usefulness in the following disorders:

- Schizophrenia
- Substance Abuse
- Bipolar Disorder
- Eating Disorders
- Criminal Behavior
- Anger and Aggression

There are even more indications for the use of CBT that I will not mention at this time.

CBT STRUCTURE

The classical structure of a CBT program includes a certified CBT therapist, 30 to 60-minute counseling sessions, weekly or biweekly sessions, and homework. The person being counseled will be expected to continue their therapy by performing a series of cognitive exercises between sessions at home. The "homework" extends the therapy session and advances the process of neuroplasticity.

CBT is not structured to be a lifetime of counseling. The goal is to teach a person how to interrupt maladaptive thinking. Once taught the need for continued counseling is finished. The individual becomes their own counselor and may only need occasional "refresher" sessions. The sessions continue until the goal of retraining has been met. As was mentioned earlier in this chapter, CBT invokes "neuroplasticity." The process takes time (demonstrable neuroplasticity has been shown on functional MRI testing as early as six weeks). The patient will need to be patient and do their homework for the "neuroplasticity" to occur.

Secret Number 3: Not all counselors that advertise themselves as CBT therapists are actually trained in it.

THE CBT COUNSELOR

Not all counselors that market themselves as a "CBT Therapist" are actually trained in the modality. When CBT was first developed, there were few therapists. Today most Americans will have access to this very effective form of therapy. There are some on-line programs available too. When attempting to find the right therapist remember to inquire about their training in CBT and see how the "personality fit" is with them. When it comes to a psychotherapist, the emotional bond that you develop is essential for the therapy to be effective.

IN CONCLUSION

I have discussed the neurophysiology, indications, and structure of Cognitive Behavioral Therapy. This therapy is an effective way to reduce pain and treat a variety of disorders. You will need to check and see if your insurance will cover this form of therapy as not all do. This form of therapy should be an adjunct to most people with chronic pain.

III. Biofeedback Therapy Secrets

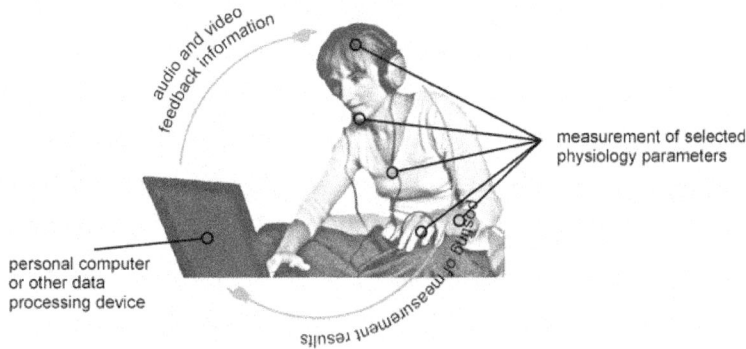

Biofeedback Therapy (BT) is defined as willful modulation of an automatic biologic process. As BT has no appreciable side effects, it would be an excellent choice for chronic pain treatment. The application of this mode of therapy does not require a medical degree, is safe, is simple, and can be administered at home.

Secret Number 1: Biofeedback uses willful control of automatic physiologic functions to reduce pain.

THE NEUROPHYSIOLOGY OF BIOFEEDBACK THERAPY

Pain is mediated by all three segments of the nervous system: the peripheral, central, and autonomic nervous systems. Proportionate participation of each system is dependent on whether the pain is acute or chronic. Acute pain is defined as pain that lasts for less than three months. Acute pain is adaptive and gives evidence of a disturbance existing in a complex biologic organism. Indeed, the absence of the ability to feel pain (there are acquired and inherited diseases that can do this) shortens life expectancy in the individuals that suffer from such maladies. Chronic pain is defined as continuous or daily pain that lasts for more than three months. Chronic pain is maladaptive and increases mortality as a separate risk factor. The presence of chronic pain shortens human life expectancy and requires effective treatment.

Biofeedback is particularly useful in chronic pain syndromes. In chronic pain, central mediating mechanisms are the predominate generator for the pain. This is not true of most acute pain. Biofeedback Therapy is not as useful for acute pain therefore. Through BT, central sensitization (where the nervous system increases the efficiency of pain transmission), autonomic pain mediation, hormonal up regulation, and neurotransmitter up regulation are all affected. By influencing automatic biologic processes with BT all the aforementioned processes are "turned down." The resultant effect is a reduction in chronic pain.

BT modulates the transmission, perception, and generation of pain. BT techniques simply make that which is automatic in human physiology noticeable to the individual and subject to the will. This is called "operationalizing" an automatic process. BT requires a device to learn how to accomplish this. By employing mental exercises, the patient learns how to effect changes in automatic physiologic processes that are being monitored by an electronic device.

THE STRUCTURE OF BIOFEEDBACK TECHNIQUE

Secret Number 2: Biofeedback requires the use of an electrical device to measure an automatic physiologic process.

By measuring heart rate, muscle tension, temperature, and skin perspiration (all physiologic functions that are usually automatic), an individual can be taught how to affect a change in these processes through mental imagery. The effect is to down regulate pain in many cases. After several BT sessions (usually 10) an individual can often forego the use of the BT machine and employ the same relaxation or mental imagery that was used to affect the targeted automatic response.

There are four basic biofeedback machine training tools:

1) Galvanic Skin Response Training:

By measuring the conductivity of the skin to a gentle electrical current, an indirect measure of the skin sweating can be assessed. Modulation of this automatic function with BT would help treat anxiety and its effect on pain.

2) Electro-Myographic Response Training:

By measuring the muscle reactivity to a gentle electrical current, an indirect measure of muscle reactivity can be assessed. Modulation of this automatic function with BT would help treat muscle spasm and muscle pain.

3) Heart Rate Response Training:

By modulating heart rate with BT, reduction of the effect of stress on pain can be accomplished.

4) Skin Temperature Response Training:

By modulating finger temperature with BT, reduction of the effect of stress on pain can be accomplished.

271 | P a g e

Note that each of the above measuring tools are measuring body metrics that are usually automatic. Through relaxation techniques and mental imagery, the effect on the metric can have a physiologic effect on the chronic pain that is being treated.

BIOFEEDBACK INDICATIONS

The following disorders have been shown to benefit from BT:

- Chronic Low Back Pain
- Fibromyalgia
- Chronic Temporomandibular Joint Dysfunction
- Chronic Abdominal Pain
- Chronic Headaches
- Hypertension
- Chronic Urinary Incontinence
- Chronic Fecal Incontinence
- Chronic Anxiety
- Phantom Limb Pain

The following conditions may be helped with BT:

- ADHD (Attention Deficit Hyperactivity Disorder)
- COPD (Chronic Obstructive Pulmonary Disease)
- Raynaud's Disease
- Chronic Constipation
- Asthma

- Epilepsy
- Rheumatoid Arthritis

Secret Number 3: There are no dangerous side effects to Biofeedback Therapy.

BIOFEEDBACK TREATMENT FREQUENCY

Because of the complexity of the nervous system and its uniqueness in each individual, a standard prescription of BT for everyone is not possible. Each individual will need to utilize the BT technique as recommended by their primary care practitioner. It may take up to 10 sessions before a reduction in pain is observed. Some conditions require many more sessions before a benefit is observed (reduction in blood pressure may take 20 sessions). Each session usually lasts 30 minutes.

IN CONCLUSION

It will take some patience on your part. Best results are seen when the treatments are guided by a trained technician in BF. Keep an open mind and commit to at least 10 treatments before deciding to continue with the treatment or not. As always, check and make sure your medical insurance carrier covers this type of therapy. BT can be a very effective adjunctive therapy in chronic pain.

IV. Magnesium Supplementation Secrets

Symptoms of magnesium deficiency

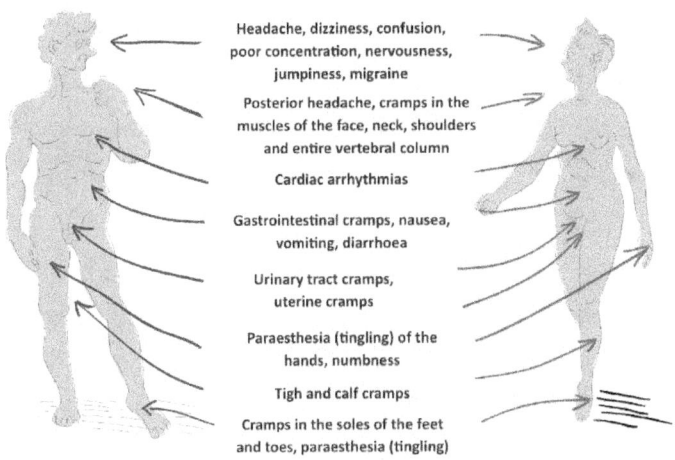

Magnesium is involved in more than 300 enzymatic reactions in the human body. It is vital in the normal function of muscles, the heart, the brain, the kidneys, the gastro-intestinal tract, blood vessels, nerves, immune system, and bones.

This section will concentrate on magnesium for pain and the syndromes that are best suited for treatment with supplementation. The wide range of physiologic participation by magnesium requires that we restrict our discussion to the pain syndromes.

THE PHYSIOLOGY OF MAGNESIUM

Secret Number 1: Magnesium is necessary for overall body health.

A brief discussion on how magnesium actually works will lead to a deeper understanding of why magnesium for pain is such an effective treatment. The physiology of the human body (how it works) is intimately related to the concentrations of charged particles called ions. The distribution of these charged particles across a cell membrane create voltage (like a battery) that electrically drives human physiology. Generally, certain charged particles tend to collect on the inside of cells while other charged particles collect on the outside (though the same particles can be found both inside and outside the cell). This creates "a tension" for any given particle to want to move where there are less (no collection). This is called a concentration gradient and a voltage potential.

The human body efficiently powers chemical reactions by creating numerous gradients throughout the body. The resulting reactions are very energy efficient and keep the operating temperature of the human body at 98.6 degrees Fahrenheit. Otherwise, the human body would operate at a much higher temperature than it does in health.

Magnesium is the second most important positively charged ion inside the human cell (the first being Potassium). It is the "first cousin" to Potassium. Where you find Potassium you usually find Magnesium (MG). Magnesium can be found in bone, muscle, soft tissue, and blood. The majority of MG is in bone (53%). Since MG is mostly "inside," the actual blood level of MG is a crude measurement of the actual amount of MG within a human body. MG deficiency can occur even though the blood level is normal.

Secret Number 2: Magnesium exerts its therapeutic effect by participating in cell membrane electrical balance.

MG cannot be manufactured by the human body. It is taken in from certain high MG containing foods. MG is absorbed from the ileum and colon. From there it is mostly protein bound and carried by the bloodstream to be distributed throughout the body. Excess MG is excreted by the kidneys. MG treats a host of disorders as previously stated.

INDICATIONS FOR MAGNESIUM SUPPLEMENTATION

The following disorders are particularly well treated by MG supplementation:

1) *Migraine Headaches (MH):*

MH are a type of a severe headache characterized by severe, throbbing pain on one side of the head. The first onset of MH usually begins around puberty with most cases having a family history of MH. Women are more prone to MH. MHs also are associated with visual changes just prior to the headache (called visual scotoma). Scotoma are often described as vision that "is as if looking through a broken mirror." Nausea and vomiting are also very commonly associated symptoms.

One of the mechanisms of generation of a MH is thought to be spasm of the blood vessels in and around the brain. MG is an obvious choice for treatment as it causes smooth muscle relaxation (arteries have smooth muscle in the wall). An acute MH can be stopped by the administration of intravenous MG. To prevent MH, daily dosing with oral MG has been shown to decrease the frequency and intensity of MH.

2) Fibromyalgia (FM):

FM is a complex disorder of chronic muscle and joint pain. Examination of the painful areas is noteworthy for pain to palpation of "trigger point" areas. Microscopic analysis of these areas reveals no anatomic abnormality. The syndrome is thought to be mediated by a central nervous system abnormality along with metabolic abnormalities within muscle cells. Supplemental MG in patients with FM has shown some beneficial effects. The oral form of MG taken daily may reduce some of the diffuse aches that occur in FM.

3) Osteoarthritis (OA):

There are many forms of arthritis. The most common form is Osteoarthritis. Several studies have shown that MG oil applied to the skin over affected joints can significantly reduce the pain of OA.   The mechanism seems to be a competitive inhibition of Calcium and its effect on modulating pain through a neurotransmitter called NMDA. The MG competes with Calcium and stops pain transmission. There may also be an anti-inflammatory effect of the MG.

Secret Number 3: Oral dosing of magnesium can have systemic benefits but is also associated with diarrhea more commonly than other forms of magnesium.

MAGNESIUM DOSING

The following dosing regimens have been used in therapy:

1) For Migraine Headaches:

The most common dose for MH as a prevention seems to be 600mg twice a day. You should start with a lower dose and gradually increase the dose for headache relief to avoid the side effect of diarrhea. Not all forms of MG taken orally are absorbed the same. MG is best taken with food to increase its absorption and decrease diarrhea. For an acute headache, an intravenous dose of MG can be used and should only be given in an acute care setting due to the possible side effects of cardiac arrhythmia.

2) For Fibromyalgia:

There is no specific dose for FM. Most authors seem to recommend starting at a low dose and gradually increasing the dose until the symptoms are relieved or side effects occur. As previously stated, one form of MG may not work. You may need to try several different preparations before relief is achieved.

3) For Osteoarthritis:

Although the chelated form of MG has been touted as better for arthritis, there are no studies that actually support this. You could start with the lowest dose by mouth and gradually increase until relief or side effects are achieved. The more usual form of therapy recommended by authors is the MG Oil preparations. These are applied to the areas of pain after showering. The oil is allowed to be absorbed and reduction of symptoms is observed. The oil is applied according to the duration of relief. Absorption is not an issue as the MG is absorbed through the skin. Diarrhea is also less frequent with this mode of administration.

SIDE EFFECTS OF MAGNESIUM

Because of the many enzymatic effects of MG (over 300 different reactions) an excess level of MG has a diverse array of symptoms related to the organ systems that utilize MG in their enzymatic processes. Skeletal muscles, heart, brain, kidneys, gastro-intestinal tract, blood vessels, nerves, immune system, and bones can all be affected with excess MG. Usually, excess MG is excreted by the kidneys. For that reason, MG side effects more commonly occur in people with kidney disease. If you or a loved one is taking MG be sure that you do not have underlying kidney disease.

Diarrhea is the most common side-effect of Magnesium supplementation. For this reason, the Magnesium oil is preferred over the oral dosing. However, in cases of diffuse pain the oral form is used. If using the oral form, starting with a low dose and increasing until pain relief or diarrhea is recommended.

IN CONCLUSION

I have reviewed the physiology, uses, doses, and side effects of MG supplementation. Magnesium supplementation may reduce chronic pain and is associated with very few side effects when kidney function is normal. Have your primary care provider supervise your use of magnesium for chronic pain.

V. Counter-irritant Skin Cream Therapy (Australian Dream) Secrets

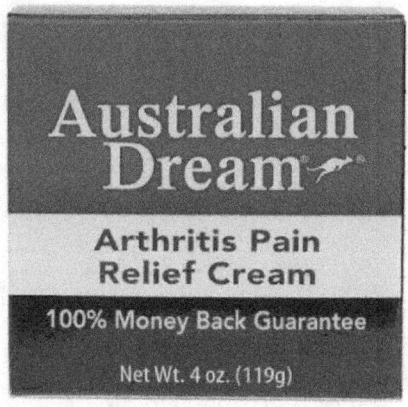

So there I was...watching a favorite show on TV (taking a break from creating posts for my websites) and a man with the kindest sort of smile, Chuck Woolery, does a commercial for Australian Dream. He states that the cream is effective for the relief of minor aches and pains. Chuck goes on to state that the company for this product has an "empty jar" money back guarantee. If anyone uses the entire jar and does not obtain relief all they have to do is send back the empty jar to get a full refund.

Secret Number 1: Australian Dream has ingredients that can provoke an allergic reaction. Highly allergic people should be cautious using this OTC cream.

THE INGREDIENTS OF AUSTRALIAN DREAM

Australian Dream is a cream that is applied to the skin for minor aches and pains. It is actually not from Australia nor is it sold there. It is manufactured by an unnamed company in Florida. Nature's Health Connection is the labeling (marketing) company, which distributes the cream. "Australian Dream" has inactive as well as active ingredients. They are listed as follows:

INACTIVE INGREDIENTS

Ingredient Name

TRIDECETH-6 (UNII: 3T5PCR2H0C)

WATER (UNII: 059QF0KO0R)

EMU OIL (UNII: 344821WD61)

POTASSIUM SORBATE (UNII: 1VPU26JZZ4)

EDETATE SODIUM (UNII: MP1J8420LU)

.ALPHA.-TOCOPHEROL ACETATE (UNII: 9E8X80D2L0)

BUTYLENE GLYCOL (UNII: 3XUS85K0RA)

DIMETHYL SULFOXIDE (UNII: YOW8V9698H)

C13-14 ISOPARAFFIN (UNII: E4F12ROE70)

ETHYLHEXYL STEARATE (UNII: EG3PA2K3K5)

GLUCOSAMINE SULFATE (UNII: 1FW7WLR731)

LAURETH-7 (UNII: Z95S6G8201)

METHYLISOTHIAZOLINONE (UNII: 229D0E1QFA)

ACTIVE INGREDIENT/ACTIVE MOIETY

Ingredient Name	Basis of Strength	Strength
HISTAMINE DIHYDROCHLORIDE (UNII: 3POA0Q644U) (HISTAMINE - UNII:820484N8I3)	HISTAMINE DIHYDROCHLORIDE	0.025 g in 100 g

The inactive ingredients presumably have no medicinal value. They are utilized in the cosmetic industry to provide a pleasing aroma, a smooth texture, and as a vehicle to evenly suspend the therapeutic substance for skin application. Skin reacts to oils, creams, and gels differently. Generally, an oily preparation hydrates skin making it softer. Oils also are a bit messy and can mark clothing. Creams are less hydrating but will usually not stain clothing. Gels actually dry the skin surface leaving it "flakey." Many manufacturers use creams as a nice intermediate carrier for their therapies.

Histamine Dihydrochloride is the active ingredient in Australian Dream. It was originally used as an injectable medicine in the treatment of a specific type of leukemia. As a topical agent (applied to the skin) it works as a "rubifacient." Rubifacients cause the skin to become reddened enlarging small surface blood vessels. This causes a warming sensation in the area where the cream is applied (most people find this painless).

THE THERAPEUTIC MECHANISM OF AUSTRALIAN DREAM

By stimulating the skin, a complex sensory reflex is stimulated that sends neural signals back to the spinal cord. In the spinal cord, the transmission of pain is diminished by the spinal reflex. Subsequently, the perception of pain is diminished and a person feels less pain.

Secret Number 2: Australian Dream works by a counter-irritative mechanism.

This is the mechanism whereby most over-the-counter pain relieving skin therapies work. It is not by their direct absorption into the bloodstream but by their "counter-irritative" effect. This is similar to many other pain relieving therapies such as hot packs, cold packs, and even acupuncture. The mechanism is quite complex and was described by Drs. Melzack and Wall in 1965. They coined the term "Gate Theory" for pain modulation in the spinal cord. Their description of the spinal cord pain transmission was like that of a gate. If you "close the gate" you don't let the pain transmission through. Counter-irritants or rubifacients probably work through a similar mechanism.

Benefits:

- Cheap relative to other prescription medications
- Safe as it is not ingested
- Easy to use as it is applied to the skin
- Over-the-counter so you do not have to obtain a Doctor's prescription to use it
- Readily available in stores and on-line
- Has a "jar back" guarantee
- Is made in the U.S.
- The company has an excellent Better Business Bureau rating

PRECAUTIONS AND SIDE EFFECTS OF AUSTRALIAN DREAM

Here is a listing of precautions when using Australian Dream:

- *The active ingredient may cause a skin reaction that can evoke allergic symptoms due to the histamine dihydrochloride.* Histamine is a key substance in acute allergic reactions. If a person is highly allergic they will want to be very careful using this substance. If you are thinking to use it, you may want to put a small amount on your arm to see if you react to it first.

- Notice that in the "inactive ingredient" list chondroitin is listed. The source for the chondroitin is shellfish. If you have a shellfish allergy (quite common), you may have a significant allergic reaction to this cream.

- Because of the "counter-irritative" effect you must avoid getting the cream in your eyes.

- Caution is recommended in pregnant women (I could find no explanation for this).

- Placing the cream onto an open wound is also not recommended (the cream then gets absorbed into the blood stream).

- Tightly wrapping the area after the cream is applied is also not recommended (presumably this would increase the skin irritation too much).

Secret Number 3: The use of Australian Dream in pregnancy is not recommended.

IN CONCLUSION

Because of the allergic symptoms that can be evoked with this product I advise caution for people who have a strong history of allergies. As always, you should use this therapy under the guidance of your primary care provider. You may find pain relief with this cream and other creams in the category of "counter-irritants." They are useful for more mild forms of chronic pain.

VI. Bioelectrical Therapy Secrets

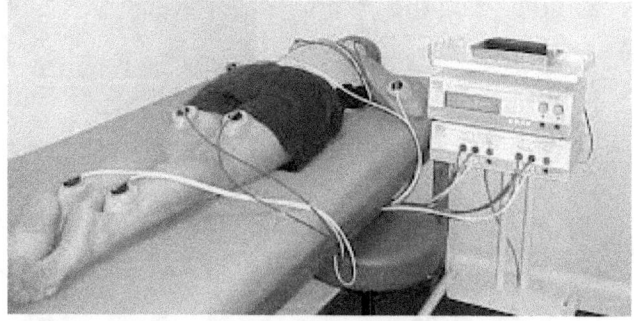

What does it mean to you when I say "Bio-electrical Therapy?" Perhaps it conjures up images of "electro-shock therapy" or some slick marketing presentation by a scammer? In the past you would have been right to have been wary of this form of therapy. The fact is the use of electricity for chronic pain has been a curiosity for centuries. There are anecdotal reports of people being struck by lightning (surviving of course) and their chronic pain completely resolving. There have also been people with incurable cancers being struck by lightning and having complete resolution of their cancers.

After all, isn't the human body electrical? It is indeed, and it would make sense that electrical current could be applied in some therapeutic sense. But how...how much...in what form? The actual scientific studies had been few up to fairly recently. *I will be specifically discussing one form of bioelectrical therapy called Horizontal Therapy (HT). It is a form of electrical therapy that targets cell membrane polarities horizontally and selectively stimulates an action potential.* The stimulation comes from using dual frequency electrical waves (one below the action potential threshold and one above it). An action potential is a sudden shift of electrical charge across a cell membrane.

Secret Number 1: The physiology of the human body uses a combination of biochemical and bioelectrical energy to power its systems.

THE PHYSIOLOGY OF BIOELECTRICAL THERAPY

Nearly all active human tissues utilize a bioelectric or biochemical energy based system. Each system is powered by polar electric charges that open and close chemical receptors (a receptor is a designated "parking spot" for a chemical), stimulate depolarization (depolarization is where the membrane electrical charge shifts), and can open or close a cell membrane channel (like the gate in a castle wall).

What makes Horizontal Therapy (HT) unique from other electrical therapies is the ability to modulate frequency (how many waves pass over a spot in a period of time) and amplitude (how large the waves are) to treat certain disorders specifically. It is well known that "one size does not fit all" for therapies so that the ability to adjust the electrical wave in Horizontal Therapy makes it very useful in a variety of disorders. Since healing utilizes multiple chemical messengers and cell types, Horizontal therapy can be used to augment this process (such as the healing of fractured osteoporotic vertebrae). Furthermore, the muscle relaxation that is generated by HT not only relaxes voluntary muscle but also involuntary (such as found in large blood vessels).

Secret Number 2: HT requires trial and error to find the best electrical prescription for any given patient for any given disorder.

INDICATIONS FOR HORIZONTAL THERAPY

The following conditions have been shown to
be benefited by HT. *Remember that HT works for some
people and not others. The reason for this is not exactly
known but may be due to specific individual electrical
frequency differences between human beings.*

- Migraine Headaches
- Carpel Tunnel Syndrome
- Acute and Chronic Back Pain
- Acute and Chronic Tendonitis
- Sciatica
- Acute and Chronic Neck Pain
- Acute and Chronic Hand Pain
- Post-Surgical Pain
- Plantar Fasciitis
- Acute and Chronic Elbow Pain
- Acute and Chronic Shoulder Pain
- Acute and Chronic Knee Pain
- Acute and Chronic Ankle Pain
- Neuropathic Pain

HORIZONTAL THERAPY PRECAUTIONS

Due to the electro-stimulatory effect of HT the following
conditions are not recommended for HT use:

- Pregnancy

- Blood Clotting Disorders
- People with electrical devices implanted or attached to them
- People who have responded adversely to electro-therapy of a different type
- People who have electrical field sensitivity
- Poorly controlled epilepsy

Secret Number 3: HT should not be used in pregnancy as it may induce labor.

IN CONCLUSION

HT is a very low risk, effective treatment for a variety of pain disorders. The "electrical prescription" from person to person may differ substantially. This would mean that some degree of trial and error will be required to find the best frequency and amplitude for each person.

VII. Lyrica (Pregabalin) Secrets

There is no possible way to treat chronic pain without risk to the person experiencing it. Nearly all the medicinal therapies on the market today can offer some relief while also carrying with them some threat. This section will be my critical appraisal of the use of Lyrica for nerve pain. If you have never experienced neuropathic pain (pain that originates from a dysfunction of the nervous system) or never knew of someone with it then you may not realize how difficult it is to treat.

BASIC NEUROPHYSIOLOGY

Finding medications that are effective for this type of pain has been very challenging for medical researchers. Neuropathic pain has an ability to change with time. The nervous system is not a system of wires that is developed as a child and remains fixed. It is actually a system that is constantly changing and adapting to internal and external stimuli.

Our nervous system not only changes its function (like a reactive software program) but also changes its structure. Can you imagine a computer that could "rewire" itself or reconstruct the microchip processor in response to the way you use it? That would give the type of change that occurs in the nervous system with neuropathic pain.

Because of this "adaptability" of the nervous system (called neuroplasticity) it is a "moving target" for medical researchers. It is very difficult to construct a scientific study on something that is constantly changing. Furthermore, the stimuli that induce change in the nervous system are not only external but internal too. The very thoughts that we have can affect our nervous system as if we performed the action in the physical (not just in our mind). So when a person imagines playing the piano their brain actually fires in the same electrical pattern as if they were playing the piano in real time. It stands to reason that a medicine that treats neuropathic pain will affect not only the physical but also the mental aspects of pain.

THE MECHANISM OF LYRICA

Lyrica (trade name) or pregabalin (generic name) is a synthetic substance that was developed and marketed by the Pfizer drug company. *It is the first medicine to be officially approved in the United States by the FDA for primary use in the treatment of neuropathic pain states.* All other medicines that were used for neuropathic pain, before the development of Lyrica, were used as "off-label" treatment for neuropathic pain with the hope that they might work. *Lyrica was the first medicine developed that proved it is consistently effective for neuropathic pain.*

Secret Number 1: Lyrica works non-specifically on nerve cells through a GABA mechanism.

The chemical structure of Lyrica closely resembles a naturally occurring chemical messenger found in the nervous system called GABA (gamma-amino butyric acid). GABA modulates pain by reducing the generation and transmission of pain signaling. It is what is called an inhibitory neurotransmitter for pain. When a person takes Lyrica the levels of GABA go up in the nervous system. This reduces the generation and transmission of pain. This is the good part about this medication.

Unfortunately, Lyrica does not just affect pain nerve cells but other nerve cells too. The inhibitory effect on other areas of the nervous system "sets Lyrica up" to cause a wide range of side effects. Furthermore, due to the highly individualized nature of the nervous system (every human being is so unique), the predictability of who will suffer major side effects is difficult.

LYRICA INDICATIONS

The use of Lyrica has been applied in the following three circumstances:

1) *In the treatment of neuropathic pain:*

- Neuropathic pain caused by Diabetes Mellitus.
- Neuropathic pain caused by "Shingles"
- Neuropathic pain caused by a host of other illnesses

2) *In the treatment of certain types of seizures*

3) In the treatment of Fibromyalgia

Secret Number 2: Lyrica has both on label and off-label uses.

It is also very common for Doctors to use medications like Lyrica for "off-label" indications. This means using it for disorders that may be helped with the medication but are not officially approved for use by the FDA. Many common medications are used in this manner and it does not mean the Doctor is "experimenting."

LYRICA DOSING

Lyrica is begun at a low starting dose, taken by mouth, and given two or three times per day. Each starting dose is different based on the disorder being treated, the size of the individual, and other body functions that are taken into account by the prescribing practitioner. After the starting dose has been taken for several weeks (Lyrica does not relieve pain immediately like an opiate based medicine does) the person taking the medication is re-evaluated by the prescriber. A dose adjustment is made to improve pain relief and reduce side effects.

This adjustment process may go on for many weeks or months before an "optimal dose" is achieved. An "optimal dose" would be one which has a significant relief of pain with a minimum of side effects. It requires much patience on the part of a person who is already experiencing pain. Lyrica is not indicated for acute pain. Often times other medications will need to be added in order that the person with pain can "hold out" until the Lyrica begins to work.

Secret Number 3: Lyrica is often started simultaneously with an opiate pain medicine as it may take several weeks for the Lyrica to begin to work.

SIDE EFFECTS OF LYRICA

Lyrica works on many types of nerve cells. Because of this there are many side effects that can be induced by Lyrica:

- Dizziness in 30%
- Sleepiness in 20%
- Dry Mouth in 15%
- Edema in 16%
- Visual Changes in 13%
- Accidents in 11%

In addition to the numerous side effects of Lyrica, there are also over 604 different drugs that Lyrica interacts with. Of the 604 drugs, 27 of the drugs have 6 major different types of interactions. The remainder of interactions are classified as "minor." Because of what has been said, every person taking Lyrica needs to be carefully evaluated for potential side effects and drug interactions. Starting a person on Lyrica requires careful evaluation, thorough instructions, and close follow-up by a medical practitioner experienced in the use of this substance.

Though there are other medications for neuropathic pain, none have been as consistently effective as Lyrica. Here are a few over the counter alternatives:

- Alpha Lipoic Acid
- Omega-3-Fatty Acids
- Primrose Oil
- Acetyl-L-Carnitine

Notice that I have not given the doses or how to take these alternative medications. You will need to discuss beginning any new therapies with your medical practitioner.

IN CONCLUSION

I have discussed neuropathic pain, what Lyrica is, how it works, when to use it, dose, and possible side effects. *Despite the long list of side effects and interactions, Lyrica can be used safely under the supervision of a medical practitioner.* I observed several very dramatic improvements with neuropathic pain in patients who were placed on Lyrica in my Pain Management practice. It is essential that close follow-up occurs with the primary care provider when a patient is placed on this medicine. The pain relief from this medicine can be miraculous.

VIII. Cymbalta Secrets

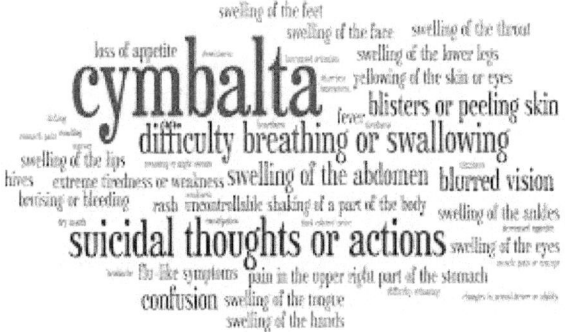

Did you know that chronic pain and depression are closely linked? People with chronic pain as their primary disorder often report the development of depression. Furthermore, people with depression as their primary disorder report more complaints of chronic pain. This section will be a review of Cymbalta as a pain medication.

THE NEUROPHYSIOLOGY OF CYMBALTA

The neurochemistry of chronic pain and depression is closely related. Similar neurotransmitters (the brain chemicals responsible for nerve signal transmission) are utilized by the brain for chronic pain and depression. I like to think of chronic pain and depression as "first cousins." So when a doctor tells you that your pain "is all in your head" they are technically correct (though they are probably using this phraseology to keep you at "arm's length" in preparation for a psychiatric referral).

Why certain people manifest their altered brain chemistry as chronic pain instead of depression is an area of active clinical research at the present time (as is the reverse). It seems that very creative people (with highly active associative cortex brain function) have a much greater likelihood of developing depression (think Vincent Van Gough). Finally, people who are depressed, who develop a physical condition that results in chronic pain, report more intense levels of pain than those people who have a similar chronic pain condition without depression.

So you can see that depression and chronic pain are inextricably linked. By the way, this does not mean that your chronic pain is imaginary or that the chronic pain patient is a "head job" (demeaning descriptive phraseology that does not belong in the vocabulary of anyone involved in health care).

Cymbalta (trade name) or Duloxetine (generic name) is an anti-depressant that works on the areas of the brain that modulate depression, anxiety, fibromyalgia, and neuropathic pain. It was originally developed and marketed by the Eli Lilly pharmaceutical company in 2004 (after some delay by the US FDA in regards to liver toxicity and possible cardiotoxicity). It is a Serotonin and

Norepinephrine reuptake inhibitor and is available by prescription only in most countries (definitely by prescription only in the US). It became available as generic Duloxetine in 2013.

Secret Number 1: Cymbalta recycles two neurotransmitters as the primary mechanism for its effect.

Depression is thought to occur due to an imbalance of the neurotransmitters Serotonin (ST) and Norepinephrine (NE). When either of these neurotransmitters reach critically low levels in the limbic system of the brain (the area where emotion is processed) depression can occur. Chronic pain is also mediated in similar areas of the limbic system. Here again, low levels of ST and NE are seen in people with chronic pain. Medications that elevate these transmitters will often result in the reduction of certain types of chronic pain.

Not all chronic pain is processed in the same manner. In particular, neuropathic pain (pain that comes from the dysfunction of the nervous system) is processed in the brain also using a sodium channel based mechanism. Cymbalta is particularly effective for pain relief in neuropathic conditions by blocking the sodium channel ions (Cymbalta's third mechanism of action).

Cymbalta slows down the removal ("reuptake") of NE, ST, and sodium ions from the synaptic cleft (a space between nerve cells) that transmits the nerve impulse from nerve cell to nerve cell. By allowing these transmitters to "loiter" in the synaptic cleft the nerve impulse has a greater likelihood to be transmitted. This general class of medication is called an SNRI (Serotonin and Norepinephrine Reuptake Inhibitor).

Anti-depressants that favor only blocking the reuptake of NE (TCAs-Tricyclic Antidepressants) or ST (SSRIs-Serotonin Reuptake Inhibitors) have not been found to be consistently effective for the reduction of neuropathic pain. The TCA class of antidepressants tend to be very sedating (elevated levels of NE in the brain are sedating). Whereas in the SSRI class of antidepressants, elevated levels of ST are energizing with insomnia as a major side effect.

CYMBALTA INDICATIONS

Cymbalta has been approved by the US FDA (Food and Drug Administration) for the following uses:

1) Chronic Pain from musculoskeletal conditions (in particular Osteoarthritis of the lower back).

2) Diabetic Peripheral Neuropathy (the intense burning pain in the feet seen when blood sugar is poorly controlled).

3) Fibromyalgia (a chronic pain condition where there are "trigger points" of focused pain throughout the body).

4) Generalized Anxiety Disorder (a chronic state of heightened autonomic arousal with persistent anxiety).

5) Major Depressive disorder

It has also been approved for use, in other countries, for Urinary Stress Incontinence and the peripheral neuropathy that can occur with chemotherapy. Furthermore, Cymbalta is often used by doctors in an "off-label" format. "Off-label" use of any medicine is where the medication has shown a benefit for patients but has not been officially recognized (by the FDA for instance) for such use. Many medications are used this way by physicians for their patients. Official uses for a medication are the only uses that a drug company may market. They may vary from country to country (France limits the official indications for Cymbalta as compared to the US).

Secret Number 2: Cymbalta has on label and off label uses.

CYMBALTA SIDE EFFECTS

You may expect that the dual mechanism of Cymbalta could "double" the chance of side effects. In fact, Cymbalta does have a rather impressive side effect profile. Here is a listing of the most common and severe side effects:

- Nausea/Vomiting

- Sedation

- Insomnia

- Dizziness

- Dry Mouth

- Withdrawal Syndrome: When Cymbalta is abruptly discontinued a very uncomfortable withdrawal syndrome can occur. It is characterized by "electric shock" sensations, agitation, confusion, nausea, vomiting, nightmares, and a host of other uncomfortable symptoms. A gradual reduction in dose for this medication is recommended when discontinuing it. It can take weeks to gradually wean off of Cymbalta. There is no universally accepted weaning schedule for it.

- Sexual Dysfunction: Cymbalta is well known to make it impossible to achieve orgasm in women who had no such difficulty before taking the medicine (and can also make the issue worse in women who already have a challenge in this area). Men can also be similarly affected.

- Increased Suicidality: Curiously Cymbalta, a medicine to treat depression, can actually stimulate suicidal attempts. Though this can be seen with nearly any anti-depressant, Cymbalta has received a "black box" warning for this. The US FDA attaches a "black box" warning to medications that have a proclivity for potentially serious, if not lethal, side effects.

THE ADMINISTRATION AND MONITORING OF CYMBALTA MUST BE UNDER THE SUPERVISION OF A LICENSED MEDICAL PRACTITIONER. THIS IS A POWERFUL MEDICINE THAT REQUIRES CLOSE FOLLOW-UP.

CYMBALTA DOSING

Cymbalta is generally begun at the lowest effective dose and gradually adjusted according to effect and side effects. The starting dose is generally 30 mg per day (taken once daily). It is well absorbed from the gastro-intestinal tract and primarily metabolized in the liver.

304 | P a g e

On any given dose, it takes three days for the blood level to stabilize. Therefore, dose adjustments should not be made any more frequently than every 72 hours (most doctors will adjust every one or two weeks). Doses over 120 mg per day are generally not recommended (the number of side effects at that dose may counter-balance the benefit).

Secret Number 3: Adjusting the dose of Cymbalta should not be done more frequently than every 72 hours (preferably every two weeks).

IN CONCLUSION

I have reviewed the neurophysiology, indications, side effects, and dosing for Cymbalta. This medication has been an important advance in the treatment of chronic pain (in particular neuropathic pain). Many people have had their pain significantly reduced by this medicine.

It carries with it a large responsibility for both patient and prescribing practitioner. As I have said in previous chapters in this book...the treatment of chronic pain always carries some risk. It is impossible to treat pain effectively without understanding this.

IX. Intercessory Prayer Secrets

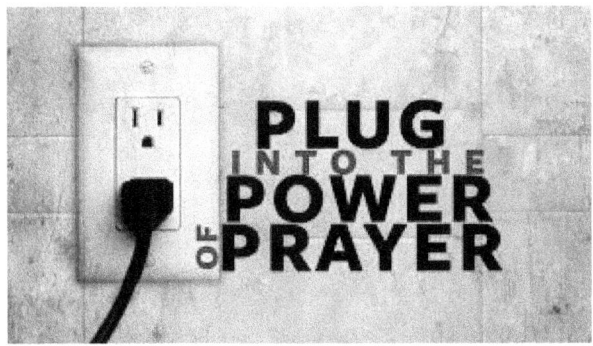

In this section, I am going to attempt to convince you why prayer for healing the sick is so essential. I became an Orthodox Christian on June 2, 1981 (I hope you don't stop reading because I said that). I remember that fateful evening when I realized that all the religious activity my parents had introduced me to was really more of an ethnic experience than true, heartfelt belief in God. I surrendered my life to Jesus Christ that night and felt the "peace that passes all understanding" for the first time in my life. I was "reborn."

MY JOURNEY

Secret Number 1: Knowing the God of Abraham, Isaac, and Jacob will make a huge difference in your life.

I was not really an atheist before that night. I just wasn't sure who God was or how to communicate with Him. I respected people of true faith. I guess I "hedged my bets" and believed that He was out there somewhere. This may sound familiar to you. My personality would not allow me to be disingenuous about this. I knew that I was on a collision course with God over this issue. At the time of my conversion I was a third-year medical student. In my relatively short time in medicine, I had already heard too many people say (when someone died), "Well, at least they are in a better place."

Ugh...well, I hope so (I would think). I mean I was not about to tell a person who was grieving that they may be wrong. Where is the compassion in doing that? After all, how does one prove or disprove God exists anyways? If I was to be true to the scientific method shouldn't I require proof for the lack of His existence? It seems some very scientific people I know require proof for His existence but not for the lack of His existence. Those of us in scientific fields believe all sorts of things that we cannot prove. I was in a quandary...that is, until June 2, 1981. That evening was such a relief. My doubts left me. My journey with Him had begun...

As I grew in faith, I was introduced to a variety of spiritual experiences that were hard to explain (rather common for spiritual experiences). As a rule, the things that I cannot explain I have trouble believing. It may be a flaw in my personality or may be what it took for me to survive the rigors of getting into and through medical school. I am not sure...all I know is that has always been my "modus operandi." Following the crowd was never my forte' either. If everyone was doing or saying the same thing, I became suspicious. My actions needed to generate from a personal belief and understanding of things. I guess that is why I was never popular (though I would have liked to have been).

When it comes to spiritual experiences, prayer had me on edge. It seemed that people of faith were always praying about something. I even had some very wonderful people tell me they were praying for me. I reasoned that, well, I need all the help I can get. I knew that the Lord prayed, His disciples prayed, very devout men and women I know pray...why am I not more committed to prayer? Then I wondered if all these people who say they believe in the power of prayer actually do? I had never personally experienced a change in outcome that could only be explained by prayer.

A REAL CASE OF HEALING BY PRAYER

I think I was in my seventh year of practice when I met Esperanza (I have changed her name to preserve her privacy). At the age of 72 years she was a vibrant lady who

308 | P a g e

worked tirelessly for her church. She had originally come into my practice when she heard me on Christian radio.

Shortly after entering my practice, Esperanza developed a swallowing problem. It seemed that certain foods "got stuck" in her throat leading her to have a very uncomfortable pressure sensation in her chest. After interviewing and examining her, I could find no obvious abnormality. She had no other complaints and felt well. I was relieved. *As a matter of protocol, I still needed to explain her swallowing problems (called dysphagia).* She was content to go no further but I insisted she go to my affiliate hospital and have a "Barium Swallow." That is an x-ray taken while swallowing a liquid mixture of barium. Usually, anything partially obstructing the esophagus will show up with that type of x-ray. I had my office staff set up the x-ray for the following week.

The next week Esperanza returned to my office with the results of her x-ray. My heart sank...the x-ray showed a baseball sized tumor at the end of her esophagus. There could be no doubt that Esperanza had Esophageal Cancer.

Telling a patient, they have a terminal illness is never easy. Many doctors find it so uncomfortable that they rush through it. Doctors are human too and telling a patient there is nothing that will change the outcome of their cancer rocks a doctor to the depths of their soul. In my practice we paused when a diagnosis like this had to be disclosed.

I entered the examination room and spoke to Esperanza:

"Esperanza I have some difficult news to tell you. You are in very deep waters…the x-ray shows you have Esophageal Cancer," I said as I tried not to break down in tears.

Esperanza said, "Does this mean I am going to die? Isn't there anything that can be done?"

I responded, "Yes, there is therapy but none of it works very well. This is an area of medicine where we have not progressed much. I know this is very hard for you Esperanza, but I will be with you every step of the way. I won't let you suffer."

Then I paused, I was overwhelmed with a thought…I need to pray with her. I have nothing else to offer her. I had recently heard my Pastor Joe Focht say during a message that God is still in the healing business. So I said to her, "Esperanza, God does not usually interrupt the laws of science that He created, but He does occasionally do so. Let's pray that He will heal you." And so I led us in prayer. I would love to be able to tell you that I prayed with confidence that the Lord would heal her. My prayer came from a heart of doubt. I knew God could do it but would He? I had never seen it and couldn't imagine it happening in Esperanza's case. I lacked faith…my prayer was very short and anemic. It was not a high lofty prayer.

Before she left, my office staff scheduled her for Upper Endoscopy (a scope that looks in the esophagus) with the Chief of Gastroenterology at my affiliate hospital. I needed a tissue biopsy of the tumor to begin her staging workup for the cancer. She thanked me for everything and left shaken…as was I.

The week went by quickly as I attended to my myriad of daily patients. On Friday, the same week I had told Esperanza of her Esophageal Cancer (four days earlier), I received a call from the Chief of Gastroenterology during the middle of my busy office hours. The conversation went like this:

Dr. Bill (the Gastroenterologist): "Hello Jeff, I finished the endoscopy on Esperanza." He was actually calling me from the endoscopy room where she was still sedated.

Myself: "How bad is it, Bill?"

He responded, "Well, I passed the scope through her esophagus, then I pulled it out, then I reinserted it, and finally I turned the scope to look up into the esophagus. Jeff, I couldn't find anything wrong. *There was no tumor present.*"

I asked, "Bill, did you see the Barium Swallow?"

He responded, "Yes, it showed a large mass which looked like Esophageal Cancer."

To which I responded, "Can you explain what happened Bill," (I knew Bill to be an agnostic)? He was silent...

It isn't the strength of our prayers or the abundance of our faith that can heal through prayer; it is the sovereign will of God that decides. *There could be no scientific explanation for a tumor that size to disappear just days after my conversation with Esperanza.* By the way, the name Esperanza translated into English means "hope."

Secret Number 2: Miraculous healings, by definition, defy scientific explanation.

AN EXPERIMENTAL STUDY OF HEALING BY PRAYER

You might be saying, "Ok Doc, so you had an isolated healing that science cannot explain. However, given enough time, science will explain everything." Does that sound familiar? I am not the only physician who has attended to a miraculous healing such as Esperanza's. There have actually been many recorded (just Google it). Because of this there has been a resurgence of interest in studying prayer from a scientific point of view. Several studies have been done to attempt to identify whether prayer is consistently effective for healing. The results have been "inconsistent." Some studies showed benefit while others show no benefit of prayer for healing. However, if you examine the studies carefully, the studies that showed no benefit had methodology that was flawed. The methodology is crucial for the scientific method.

I found one study that was very credible, used excellent methodology, and was peer-reviewed (meaning other doctors weighed in with their opinions on the study). It also had easily measured variables (so differences between groups could be quantified) and was published in a credible medical journal. It showed very significant differences between the therapy group (those prayed for) and the control group (those not prayed for).

This study compared complication rates of people in an intensive care unit. The patients that were prayed for had a much lower death rate and complication rate. The results were so astounding that the research team "crossed over" the groups. This means they stopped praying for the prayer group and started praying for the non-prayer group. What do you think happened? The death rates and complication rates of the first non-prayer group began to go down as soon as they were prayed for. The reverse happened for the first prayer group when the team stopped praying for them. Their death rate and complication rate increased soon after the team had stopped praying for them.

So that you can check out what I am saying, I have included the link to the article on prayer and healing which was published in the Southern Medical Journal in 1988:

http://europepmc.org/abstract/med/3393937

What should this mean for us when it comes to prayer as therapy for illness (especially chronic pain)?

Secret Number 3: The effect of intercessory prayer is never inconsistent or of no benefit.

PRAYER IS THE PERFECT PAIN PRESCRIPTION

If I could create a perfect therapy it would have the following features:

- It would be effective
- It would not cost a lot of money
- It would have few side effects
- It would be available "over-the-counter" and not require a prescription
- It would be effective for a wide range of illnesses
- It would be available to everyone who wanted it
- It would not be limited by the location of the people who need it

Are you "getting my drift"? If you believe in prayer, are you praying for those who need healing? If you don't believe in prayer, why not? Can anyone really justify not praying for someone who needs healing? I am actually speaking to myself when I ask those questions. I don't pray enough. Even after all the experiences and research I find myself not praying enough. Shame on me...but what about you?

IN CONCLUSION

I hope you have found this section interesting and provocative. I am not trying to make you feel badly for not praying. This was just my feeble attempt to challenge some assumptions you may have about prayer for healing the sick. *Would you really withhold a therapy that is free, is available to all, has no geographic boundaries, has no deleterious side effects, requires no prescription, and may be effective for the particular problem you are facing?* We all need to pray more for our families, our friends, and ourselves. We especially need to be praying for those who have chronic pain.

X. Hypnosis Secrets

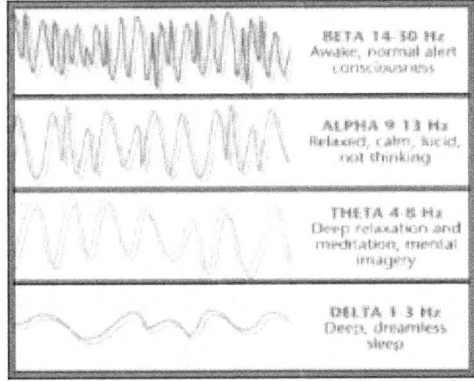

We have all seen the theatrical presentation of the hypnotist on stage who "mesmerizes" several stout looking male volunteers and gets them to do something foolish. Then...with a snap of his fingers...the men revert to normal without any memory of what just happened. That is NOT what I will be speaking to you about in this section. This section will be a scientific look at hypnosis and pain relief.

Perhaps you have several questions about hypnosis such as, "Isn't it dangerous to open my mind to a hypnotist?" Or perhaps, "Does God want me to use hypnotism as a means of therapy?" Or perhaps you have even wondered, "Will the hypnotist be able to insert thoughts into my mind that I find objectionable or distasteful?"

After reading this chapter, you will be able to answer those questions for yourself. My intention is to give you the information you need to be able to make your own decisions about therapy and "take charge" of your own pain relief.

THE NEUROPHYSIOLOGY OF HYPNOSIS

Hypnosis is an intermediate state of consciousness (called a trance in deep hypnosis), characterized by heightened susceptibility to suggestion. Not all people are prone to deep hypnosis. There is a certain type of person who will benefit the most from hypnosis. The likelihood is that their neuro-physiology (the study of the function of the nervous system) responds to hypnotic instructions for disattention (the process of the deliberate refusal to pay attention to certain things).

Secret Number 1: Hypnosis utilizes the process of disattention.

The ability to dis-attend to stimuli, both internal and external, is both genetic and an act of the will. To predict when hypnosis will have the most benefit a person must score "high" on the testing instruments that measure their suggestibility. These tests are usually administered by research clinicians who will be evaluating their hypnosis findings according to whether a study participant rates "high" or "low" on these testing instruments. However, nearly everyone with chronic pain can benefit from hypnotic therapy. Many hypno-therapists will not pre-test for suggestibility. They will simply teach the process to anyone who may benefit. Furthermore, the ability to hypnotize or self-hypnotize has been shown to improve over time. In other words, there is a training effect in how to best utilize hypnosis.

Analysis of the blood flow in certain areas of the brain has been shown to be affected with analgesic hypnosis (hypnosis that causes pain relief). The area of the brain that is most often reported is in the anterior frontal cortex (the forehead area on the surface of the brain). In people who rate "high" for hypnotic suggestion, they register an increase in the blood flow to that area of the brain as their pain decreases. Other studies have shown that the electrical activity of the brain also changes when hypnotic analgesia is occurring. A common way to measure brain electrical activity is with an Electroencephalogram (EEG). This device requires the person being hypnotized to wear electrodes applied to the skin of the head. *In people that experience hypnotic analgesia the brain wave activity tended to reflect more theta wave activity than in the people that did not experience pain relief.*

Secret Number 2: Hypnosis has measurable effects on the function of the brain.

In summary, the brain physiologic changes that have been measured are thought to be due to an increase in the inhibitory activity of the brain. This causes a reduction in the perception of the pain and subsequent reduction in measured pain.

INDICATIONS FOR HYPNOSIS

The following disorders have been shown to be positively affected by hypnotic therapy:

- In the treatment of chronic pain disorders
- In the treatment of addictions
- In the treatment of phobias
- In the treatment of sleep disorders
- In the treatment of depression
- In the treatment of post-traumatic stress disorder
- In the treatment of anger management
- In the treatment of grief
- In the treatment of obesity
- In the treatment of smoking
- In the pursuit of repressed memories

PRECAUTIONS WHEN USING HYPNOTHERAPY

There are certain precautions with hypnotic therapy. People who are prone to altered processed thinking, such as in a psychotic state, are not advised to undergo hypnosis. The hypnotic state may provoke worsening delusions or hallucinations under these circumstances. Hypnosis is also not recommended for people with active hallucinations from drugs or alcohol. Detoxification is recommended before instituting hypnotic therapy. A caveat in using hypnosis for repressed memories should also be reminded. There is a risk of "false memories" being created with deep hypnotic analysis. Finally, in people with dissociative disorders (such as multiple personality disorder), hypnotic therapy is not recommended as it may provoke spontaneous dissociation.

The hypnotic state requires a willful participation of the person involved. This precludes the likelihood of thought insertion against one's will.

Secret Number 3: Hypnosis requires willful participation to be effective.

IN CONCLUSION

I have reviewed the physiology, indications, and precautions in using hypnotic analgesia. It is very clear that this form of therapy may be very effective in reducing chronic pain in the patient that has a proclivity for hypnotic therapy.

XI. Inversion Therapy

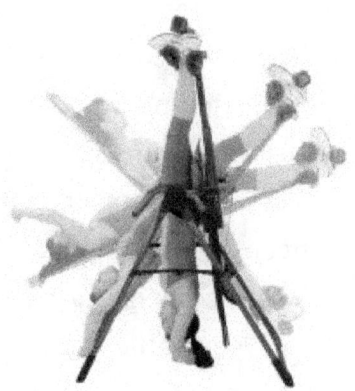

I know you have seen the commercials...a middle-aged man hanging by his ankles on a contraption that he claims has made his back pain disappear. Perhaps you were thinking, "That looks like a modern form of torture." The contraption that was being used was a type of therapy called INVERSION THERAPY. This section will be a review of the benefits of inversion therapy.

TYPES OF INVERSION THERAPY

Inversion therapy is really a form of whole body traction therapy. There are many devices that work on the same principle. There are inversion tables, inversion chairs, "anti-gravity" boots, and all the gradations in between. Many devices can be obtained for less than $100 and there are those that cost upwards of $500.

Secret Number 1: Inversion therapy is a form of traction.

The devices vary in the construction material durability, the comfort of the ankle attachment mechanism, the resting position, and the adjustability of the positions for inversion. The most intense inversion therapy is the "anti-gravity" boot device where a person is suspended vertically without any adjustment. The least intense would be the inverting chair. The inversion table is somewhere in the middle as far as intensity of traction.

MECHANISM OF ACTION

Inversion utilizes the upper part of your body as a weight for traction of the spine. The device applies the most traction to your lower back. There is some traction afforded by the weight of your head to your neck too. In this way, gravity acts to "pull apart" the tissues of the spine.

In some cases, neck and back pain comes from muscle spasm primarily. In those cases, the inversion therapy stretches the muscles, which causes reflex relaxation of the painful muscles. The effect is felt much sooner than you may expect with other disorders of the spine. In the cases, where the primary mechanism for the pain is disc degeneration pressing upon nerves in the back or neck, the relief may come much more slowly. Multiple treatments over time may be required for relief of the pain as stretching ligaments, tendons, and the disc is a slow process.

Secret Number 2: Inversion therapy requires multiple treatment sessions to be effective.

The more reversible the anatomical abnormality of the spine is the sooner the relief with inversion therapy. Most of the literature on this topic recommends that you start with an inversion angle of no more than 15 degrees. As your stamina builds, you can go to a greater degree of angle downward.

FREQUENCY OF USE

As for how many times a week and how long your sessions should be there are no universal recommendations. The old saying, "Start low and go slow" is probably wise. Therapy is also gauged by response so you should increase intensity and frequency until you see relief. After sustained relief for two weeks on a given regimen, gradually decrease the intensity and frequency to that which still maintains relief.

You also must remember that any activity that worsens your underlying cause for back pain essentially "undoes" your therapy. This may be unavoidable if you have a very physical occupation. For this reason, the timing of your therapy should be a consideration. You may want to use your inversion table when you get home from work or after a long airplane flight. *Think of your inversion therapy as if it was a medicine.* Adjust your use of it according to how you feel and your activity level. Your inversion device is your personal therapist.

INDICATIONS FOR INVERSION THERAPY

The following conditions have been found to be helped by inversion therapy:

- Chronic low back pain
- Chronic neck pain
- Neck sprain and strain
- Back sprain and strain
- Herniated Disc of the Back
- Sciatica
- Degenerative Joint Disease of the Spine
- Degenerative Disc Disease of the Spine

There may be other conditions that inversion therapy treats but the above list is the majority of the usual conditions.

PRECAUTIONS WITH INVERSION THERAPY

Inversion therapy is not for everyone. Because of the change in body position, both blood flow and breathing are affected by it. In the following conditions, inversion therapy should be used with caution or not at all:

- Morbid Obesity
- Congestive Heart Failure
- Glaucoma
- Heart Disease
- Hypertension
- Gastro-esophageal Reflux
- Hip Joint Replacement
- Knee Joint Replacement
- Ankle Disorders
- Asthma
- Chronic Obstructive Pulmonary Disease

Secret Number 3: Inversion therapy can be rigorous and must be carefully applied to people who have cardiovascular and lung disease.

THIS DISCUSSION IS NOT INTENDED TO BE MEDICAL ADVICE BUT IS INFORMATIONAL ONLY. YOU NEED TO USE INVERSION THERAPY UNDER THE DIRECTION OF YOUR PRIMARY CARE PROVIDER.

IN CONCLUSION

Inversion therapy is a useful tool for the treatment of a variety of chronic painful conditions. It is reasonably cheap, safe, and can be done at home. It will give you the flexibility to treat yourself as you need more or less therapy.

XII. Carpal Tunnel Therapy

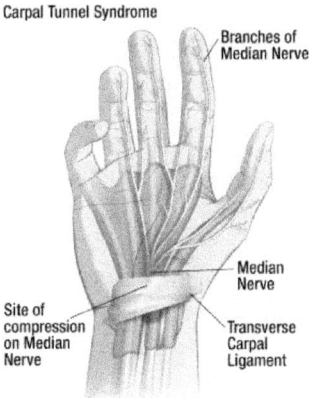

In this section, I am going to review a very common disorder of the wrist called Carpel Tunnel Syndrome or CTS and its treatment. With all the time we spend on our home computers we are all at risk for this annoying problem. I am also going to suggest a cure for carpal tunnel syndrome...and I don't mean surgery!

A REVIEW OF CARPAL TUNNEL SYNDROME (CTS)

CTS is a condition where the main nerve going into your hand is irritated or compressed. This nerve is called the Median Nerve and it accounts for 3/5 of the function of your hand. It travels through the Carpel Tunnel of your wrist into your hand. According to the Bureau of Labor Statistics, this malady is usually seen in people who repeatedly use their hands. There are over three million Americans with this condition. Women are much more commonly affected than men. It clusters in families (which means there is a genetic tendency to develop it). Furthermore, people with Diabetes Mellitus, Thyroid disease, Rheumatoid Arthritis, and Pregnancy have a higher chance of getting this annoying condition.

Secret Number 1: CTS is the most common nerve compression syndrome in America.

THE HISTORY AND PHYSICAL IN CTS

When the Median Nerve is irritated or injured, you may notice numbness, stiffness, weakness, and "tingling" pain in the wrist or hand. The pain can even radiate up the arm. There may be certain activities that make it worse like typing, using the mouse of your computer, or operating machinery that vibrates. If the symptoms go on untreated, you may develop permanent symptoms in your hand. At that point, many of the therapies that we will be discussing may not work. It is important to not ignore the symptoms. You should be evaluated by your Primary Care Physician (PCP) if these symptoms occur.

Your PCP will perform a thorough history and physical. He or she may tap on the underside of your wrist to see if a "lightning pain" is generated (called Tinel's Sign). This will mean you have CTS. For the purpose of proving the diagnosis, your PCP may order an Electromyogram/Nerve Conduction Study (EMG/NCS). It is an uncomfortable study where fine needles are pierced into your skin and a low electrical current is used to stimulate a muscle or nerve. It is not my favorite test for obvious reasons.

Secret Number 2: CTS is diagnosed by a good history and physical (not by a needle nerve conduction study).

THERAPY FOR CTS

If your History, Physical Exam, and EMG/NCS are consistent with CTS, your PCP will probably begin conservative therapy. That usually constitutes anti-inflammatory medication, a wrist splint, stretching

328 | P a g e

exercises for the wrist, and instructions on what activities to avoid.

If your symptoms persist for more than four weeks with conservative therapy, your PCP will refer you to a surgeon who specializes in a procedure called a Carpel Tunnel Release. This is a fairly simple surgery where the Transverse Carpal Ligament of the wrist is cut and the tendons compressing the Median Nerve are "released" (see the above diagram). This relieves the pressure on the Median Nerve and your symptoms usually resolve.

LIMITATIONS OF TRADITIONAL CTS THERAPY

While many people will get relief of their symptoms with these therapies, there are several drawbacks:

- Anti-inflammatories have many side-effects (i.e., stomach ulcers, kidney disease, etc.). They cause up to 17,000 deaths each year in the U.S. from Gastro-intestinal hemorrhage. These medications do nothing for the main problem in CTS...the narrow Carpal Tunnel.

- Wrist exercises may help temporarily but do not correct the main cause of the nerve entrapment...a narrow Carpal Tunnel.

- A wrist splint may help by allowing the wrist structures to rest and heal. If a splint doesn't improve your symptoms in two to four weeks, it probably isn't going to work. You see...it doesn't change the narrow Carpal Tunnel.

- Surgery will definitely enlarge the Carpel Tunnel. However, you will have to face the risk of a surgical procedure, some form of anesthesia, a permanently painful incision on your hand (60% of patients) and your symptoms may recur anyways.

AN IDEAL FORM OF TREATMENT FOR CTS

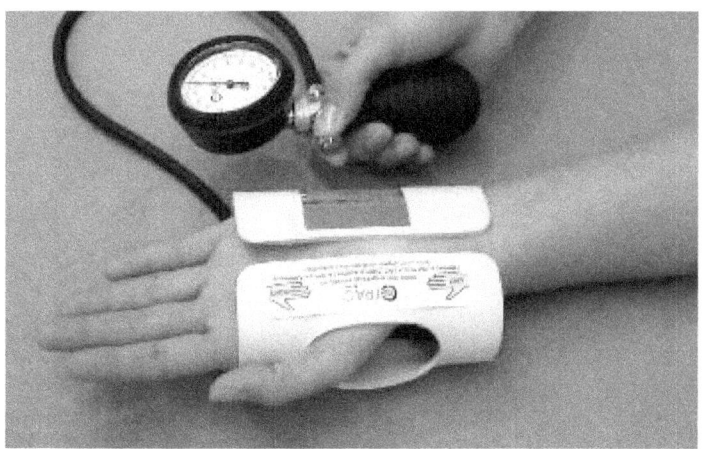

If I was going to create the perfect treatment for something I would make it effective, have few side effects, be affordable, and be able to be repeated conveniently.
There is actually a therapy that satisfies all my criteria...it is called the CTrac. The CTrac was developed in the U.S. by two Doctors who practice pain management. The device inflates on the surface of the wrist and stretches the Transverse Carpal Ligament...enlarging the Carpal Tunnel without surgery. It is worn five minutes, three times per day. Within two weeks, 70 to 80% of patients have significant relief. After using the therapy for one month, 75% of the patients no longer required surgery.

Secret Number 3: The CTrac device can be used without a needle nerve conduction study being performed. Surgery for CTS nearly always requires a needle nerve conduction study before a surgeon will operate.

IN CONCLUSION

I have reviewed the symptoms, signs, tests, and usual therapies for CTS. The CTrac is an excellent alternative to surgery. It enlarges the Carpal Tunnel without having to have a needle nerve conduction study performed and surgery. If the symptoms persist then surgery is still a viable option. However, most people can avoid surgery by repeated use of CTrac therapy.

Chapter 10 – Final Words On the Secrets Of Your Own Effective Pain Management

You have nearly reached the conclusion of the First Edition of "Secrets of Effective Pain Management."
Congratulations on your persistence. Perhaps you have noticed a pattern that emerged as you read through? I am going to review seven basic "secrets" in this last chapter. They are what I believe to be the "anchor secrets" of what I have been attempting to teach you throughout this book. These "secrets" are woven throughout the previous pages. They are the unique management concepts that my

patients, experience, and the evolving pain management literature taught me. They are as follows:

Anchor Secret Number 1: Your chronic pain is never imaginary but may seem so to those around you if its cause is not visible to them.

Remember that pain is a physiologic phenomenon. Nearly all the studies performed to diagnose the conditions that cause pain measure a structural abnormality. A person could no sooner detect the temperature of their oven by looking at it than they can detect chronic pain in another person by looking at them.

Anchor Secret Number 2: The isolation that you experience having chronic pain is not always a deliberate act of desertion on the part of your loved ones.

It can be the result of their powerlessness to help you. The combination of watching you suffer and not being able to help you is often overwhelming for people.

Anchor Secret Number 3: Empathy is essential in your pain Doctor.

How will you know if your Doctor practices this? The best way is to listen to the testimonies of patients that have already seen the pain Doctor you are planning to see. All the other available methods of identifying an empathic

Doctor on-line, in magazines, and in the newspaper are easy to falsify. Even a referral from another Doctor is not as reliable as a patient referral. A patient referral from someone you trust is the best way to find an empathic Doctor.

Anchor Secret Number 4: Diagnostic studies always have limitations in their ability to detect disease and accurately diagnose it.

Your diagnosis may require you to have several different tests performed before it is actually found. Don't give up…

Anchor Secret Number 5: The neuro-mechanism for your chronic pain is more important than the diagnosis of the disease causing it.

Over the years, I had many patients in which the diagnosis for their pain was in question but in whom I was able to relieve their pain. I do not recommend waiting for a diagnosis before relieving chronic pain (this is different from acute pain which is an early warning system).

Anchor Secret Number 6: In most cases of chronic pain there will need to be a transition to self-care.

As early as possible and as much as possible you should take the responsibility for your own pain relief. Your outcome will be much better this way and you will be less dependent on your Doctor.

Anchor Secret Number 7: There is no type or manifestation of pain that cannot be helped.

I know of patients that were told that their type of pain just couldn't be relieved (such as with Pancreatic Cancer). This is patently false. The ability to achieve relief of your pain is proportional to how aggressive your Pain Management practitioner will be. As you may expect, the more severe your pain syndrome is, the more risk there will be in relieving it.

I hope you have enjoyed this book. I need your help to improve the Second Edition. Please e-mail me with your comments, suggestions, and criticisms. I really look forward to hearing from you. My personal email is: epiduraldoc1982@gmail.com

As always, wishing you joy and healing,

Jeffrey C. Bado, D.O.

P.S.: You may want to visit my website chronicpainreliefoptions.com to learn more about what you can do to obtain relief from chronic pain. This website is updated nearly every day.

Epilogue – The Secret to Eternal Life

I have shared many secrets with you in this book. I would be remiss if I did not share my greatest secret with you. You may be wondering what motivated me to become a Pain Management physician. Yes, as I stated in the introduction to this book, seeing the suffering of my patients prompted me to go into a field I did not originally plan to practice. However, was there a deeper motivation? I believe that the type of sacrificial compassion that a Pain Doctor should have can only come from the Lord Jesus Christ. He is my ultimate example of empathy. He is the underlying motivation for my venture into the conflicted field of pain management.

I was not always a true Christian. I became one in my third year of medical school when I realized that even if a person enjoyed excellent health and was a responsible steward of their body (in other words had no bad habits) they have the same physical end as the irresponsible person. It just may take a little longer for responsible people to get there. We all will die someday. As a physician, I could see that the profession I was called to did not address the greatest issue of the living which is what about the afterlife?

The only faith on earth that answers all the fundamental questions of life is faith in Jesus Christ. Questions of human origin, meaning, morality, and destiny are definitively answered by Him. He chose to reveal this information in the most read book of all time...The Holy Bible. Through a relationship with Christ, the Word of God becomes alive. This is because He invests Himself in us by way of the Holy Spirit. When a person commits their life to Christ, a transaction occurs and God indwells the believer. No other faith makes that claim.

To qualify for this transaction between God and man you have to be one thing...a sinner. Do you qualify? Unless you have never sinned (including thoughts of sin) you qualify. That means everyone qualifies but not everyone willfully receives God's gift...Jesus Christ. It isn't that God excludes people...they exclude themselves by rejecting Him. You may think that doing good works is the way you qualify for eternal life. The problem with that approach is that it does not address your sin. A perfect God, in a perfect realm, cannot accept imperfection. But when we receive Jesus Christ His sacrifice for our imperfections...our sin...pays the price so that God can appropriate His righteousness to us. He does this in the transaction I was talking about. No other faith or belief system on earth makes this transaction.

If you have not yet received Christ as your Savior you can do so right now, as you finish this book, by praying the following prayer. Your prayer must be sincere, not simply a recitation of the words but a heartfelt belief in what you are saying. The following words will lead you into a relationship with Jesus Christ and give you eternal life:

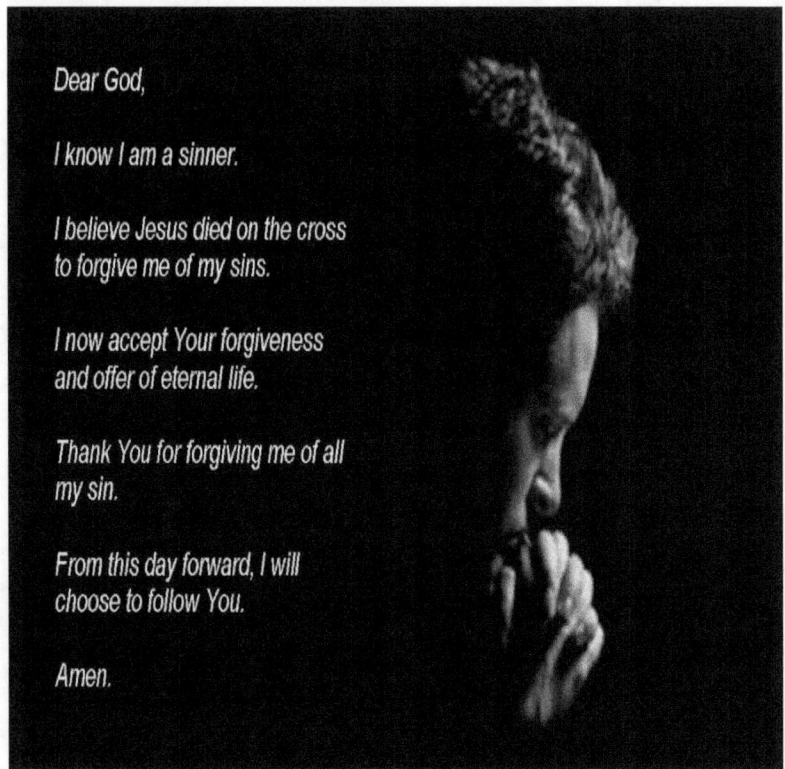

Dear God,

I know I am a sinner.

I believe Jesus died on the cross
to forgive me of my sins.

I now accept Your forgiveness
and offer of eternal life.

Thank You for forgiving me of all
my sin.

From this day forward, I will
choose to follow You.

Amen.

My friend, if you prayed that prayer sincerely God heard you and answered your prayer. I would love to know if you received Christ reading this book. You can contact me via my personal email at epiduraldoc1982@gmail.com. I will be prompt in getting back to you and have a special gift for you.

Wishing you joy and healing in Christ,

Jeffrey C. Bado, D.O.

Author

Dr. Bado is a retired General Internist, who finished his career as a full-time Pain Management physician. He is a well know physician in the Philadelphia, Pennsylvania area where he resides. His present full-time professional activity is medical writing and continually upgrading his chronic pain website: chronicpainreliefoptions.com. The focus of his medical writing is on the controversies in chronic pain management, empowering the chronic pain patient, and sharing the Gospel of Jesus Christ with anyone who will listen. If you would like to contact him he can be reached at: epiduraldoc1982@gmail.com.

www.ingramcontent.com/pod-product-compliance
Lightning Source LLC
Chambersburg PA
CBHW051440170526
45166CB00001B/61